The
Low-FODMAP
—— Solution ——

The
Low-FODMAP
Solution

Put an End to IBS Symptoms and Abdominal Pain

Cinzia Cuneo, MSc
and the Nutrition Team at SOSCuisine.com

Robert **ROSE**

For complete cataloguing information, see page 246.

Disclaimer
This book is a general guide only and should never be a substitute for the skill, knowledge and experience of
a qualified medical professional dealing with the facts, circumstances and symptoms of a particular case.

The nutritional, medical and health information presented in this book is based on the research,
training and professional experience of the authors, and is true and complete to the best of their knowledge.
However, this book is intended only as an informative guide for those wishing to know more about health,
nutrition and medicine; it is not intended to replace or countermand the advice given by the reader's personal
physician. Because each person and situation is unique, the authors and the publisher urge the reader to
check with a qualified health-care professional before using any procedure where there is a question as to
its appropriateness. A physician should be consulted before beginning any exercise program. The authors
and the publisher are not responsible for any adverse effects or consequences resulting from the use of
the information in this book. It is the responsibility of the reader to consult a physician or other qualified
health-care professional regarding his or her personal care.

The recipes in this book have been carefully tested by our kitchen and our tasters. To the best of our
knowledge, they are safe and nutritious for ordinary use and users. For those people with food or other
allergies, or who have special food requirements or health issues, please read the suggested contents of each
recipe carefully and determine whether or not they may create a problem for you. All recipes are used at the
risk of the consumer. We cannot be responsible for any hazards, loss or damage that may occur as a result of
any recipe use. For those with special needs, allergies, requirements or health problems, in the event of any
doubt, please contact your medical adviser prior to the use of any recipe.

Design and production: Kevin Cockburn / PageWave Graphics Inc.

Layout: Alicia McCarthy/PageWave Graphics Inc.

Indexer: Gillian Watts

Interior Photography: Kinga Wójcicka; except Olimpia Davies (Poached Eggs and Smoked Ham in an Orange
Sauce, Blackened Fish Fillets, Vegetable Salad with Mackerel, Provence-Style Chicken); Michael Matthew
Paynic (Egg Salad Sandwich, Chicken Salad with a Coriander-Mustard Dressing, Blue Cheese Turkey
Burgers, Bacon, Lettuce and Tomato Penne, Thai Noodles with Beef, Filet Mignon with a Creamy Paprika
Sauce, Spaghetti with Citrus and Anchovy Pesto); and Dollar Photo Club - Zoryanchik - Fotolia (Lemon
Polenta Cake)

Cover Image: Spaghetti with Citrus and Anchovy Pesto (page 152) by Michael Matthew Paynic

The publisher gratefully acknowledges the financial support of our publishing program by the Government
of Canada through the Canada Book Fund.

Canadä

Published by Robert Rose Inc.
120 Eglinton Avenue East, Suite 800, Toronto, Ontario, Canada M4P 1E2
Tel: (416) 322-6552 Fax: (416) 322-6936
www.robertrose.ca

Printed and bound in Canada

1 2 3 4 5 6 7 8 9 MI 25 24 23 22 21 20 19 18 17

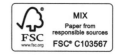

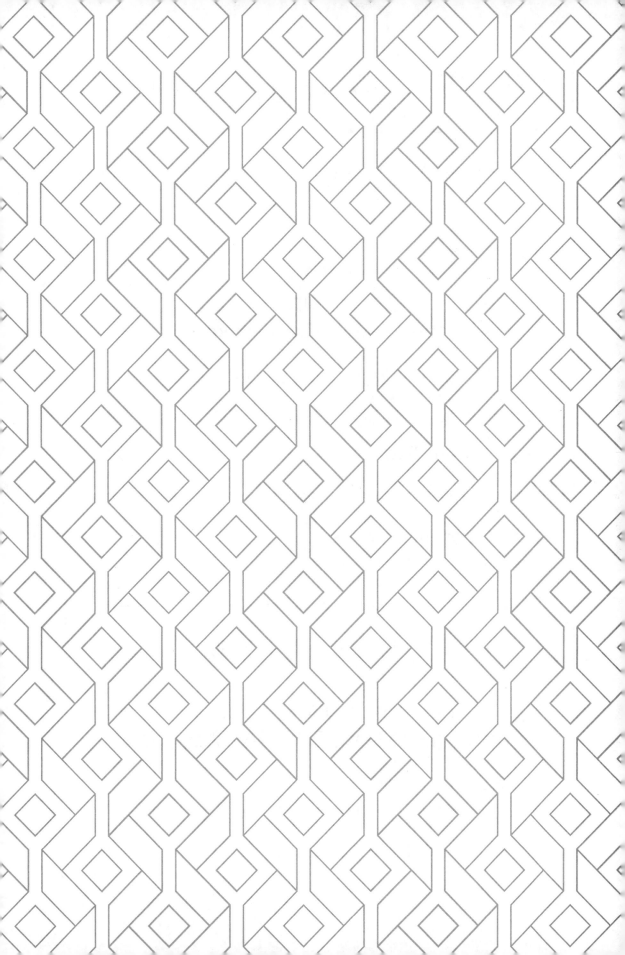

CONTENTS

PART 3
130 Healthy and Yummy Low-FODMAP Recipes

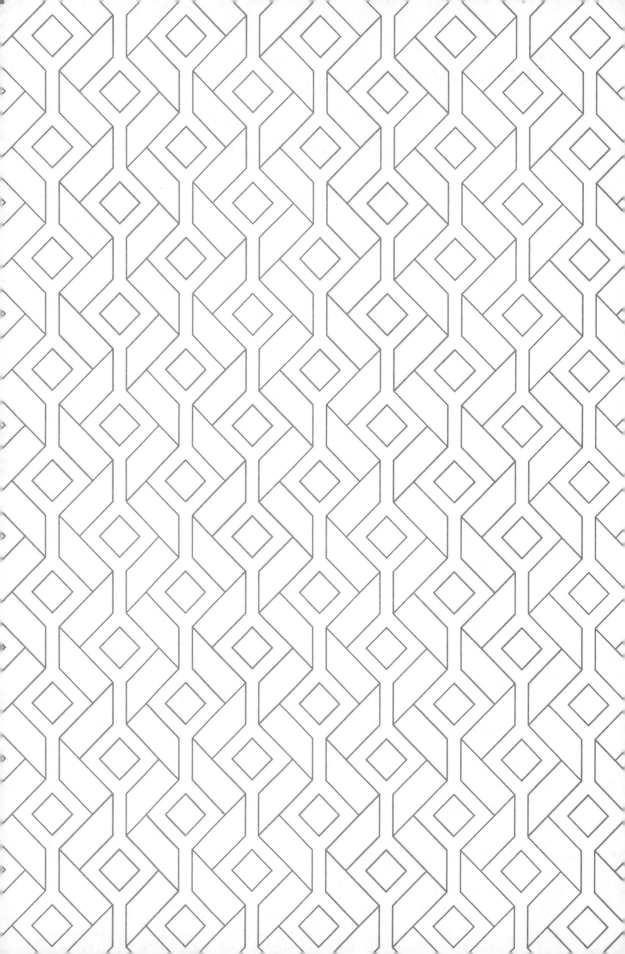

Foreword

The very first thing patients ask when they call us for gastrointestinal (GI) information is "What can I do to help this condition without taking medication?" Many patients are exasperated and exhausted after trying so many treatments without success.

In this book, SOSCuisine's dietitians make it easy to navigate through the available information about dietary options for irritable bowel syndrome (IBS). This team of highly credible dietitians has compiled diet facts based on the most recent medical literature. Of further interest to IBS patients should be SOSCuisine's helpful meal planning resources, which make including the right things in your diet — and excluding the wrong things — very easy to manage.

Do you consult the internet for health-related information? If so, you're among the 60% of Canadian web users who go online for health research. The most frequent searches are for information on specific diseases, followed by lifestyle (diet, nutrition and exercise), specific symptoms, medications, alternative therapy and surgery. As the online method of seeking information grows, so does the plethora of websites claiming accurate and up-to-date medical information. While there are many outstanding websites providing excellent and reliable guidance, it can be difficult to wade through the mishmash and separate fact from fiction.

I have been working closely with SOSCuisine as a trusted partner for several years and greatly value the information its dietitians have prepared for IBS and other gastrointestinal conditions. Since one can often have more than one health condition at a time, I am happy to recommend these quality meal plans and this excellent knowledge base for a wide range of conditions.

> SOSCuisine's helpful meal planning resources make including the right things in your diet — and excluding the wrong things — very easy to manage.

— **Gail Attara**
President, cofounder and chief executive officer, Gastrointestinal Society; president, Canadian Society of Intestinal Research

Introduction

The efficacy of a diet low in FODMAPs is increasingly being scientifically proven, and it is being used with success by tens of thousands of people around the world.

Most people who can digest any food don't know how lucky they are. The situation is rather different for millions of others who suffer from irritable bowel syndrome (IBS) and who, after each mouthful, ask themselves if they will have intestinal cramps, bloating, diarrhea or gas. This is, in effect, a daily problem for them.

About one in seven people suffers from this syndrome. However, because it relates to the intestine, a taboo subject, people rarely talk about it. The fact that the symptoms are nonspecific makes them difficult to diagnose. In addition, the available medications (antacids, antispasmodics, anti-depressants) are not effective at treating all the symptoms. Friends and family can sometimes find it hard to understand and may feel that the sufferer exaggerates his or her symptoms. As for doctors, until recently lacking effective solutions, they tended to suggest that the patient should relax. In some cases, patients are told the problem is psychological. Thus the affected person drags along with often-recurring digestive symptoms, each day and throughout life.

The last few years, the finger has been pointed at gluten and dairy as being responsible for causing several problems, including these annoying stomachaches. It is true that, when they consume less bread, pasta and dairy products, many patients tend to feel better and be less bloated. However, we now understand that this improvement is not due to the elimination of gluten and dairy, but more probably to the elimination of FODMAPs — fermentable oligosaccharides, disaccharides, monosaccharides and polyols, carbohydrates that are poorly digested in the intestine — which are found in wheat and milk, among other foods.

Fortunately, a diet low in FODMAPs is a solution that is both specific and personalized. Its efficacy is increasingly being scientifically proven, and it is being used with success by tens of thousands of people around the world.

This book's objective, therefore, is to provide you with a tool to attain intestinal well-being via a diet low in FODMAPs. This approach is effective for around 75% of those who apply it. The first part of this book presents the theory and gives you a basis to understand the logic behind this diet and its application process. The second and third parts are practical, with meal plans and recipes, and will help you apply the principles.

As a bonus, to make your task easier, on the site www.soscuisine.com you will find complete low-FODMAP meal plans tailored around your intolerances and renewed each week. The recipes are given for various portion sizes, with a shopping list, including discounts from your preferred supermarkets. It's a natural and practical way to wave goodbye to stomachaches!

Continue the Experience at SOSCuisine.com

Visit www.soscuisine.com/77880569 to access the following exclusive content:

- Our IBS/low-FODMAP support group on Facebook, moderated by a registered dietitian
- The latest news on the low-FODMAP diet
- The latest updates to the tables featured in the book, so you can benefit from the most recent findings on foods' FODMAP content
- A 20% discount on subscriptions to personalized low-FODMAP meal plans and recipes, with grocery lists
- A 10% discount on subscriptions to one-on-one coaching by a registered dietitian

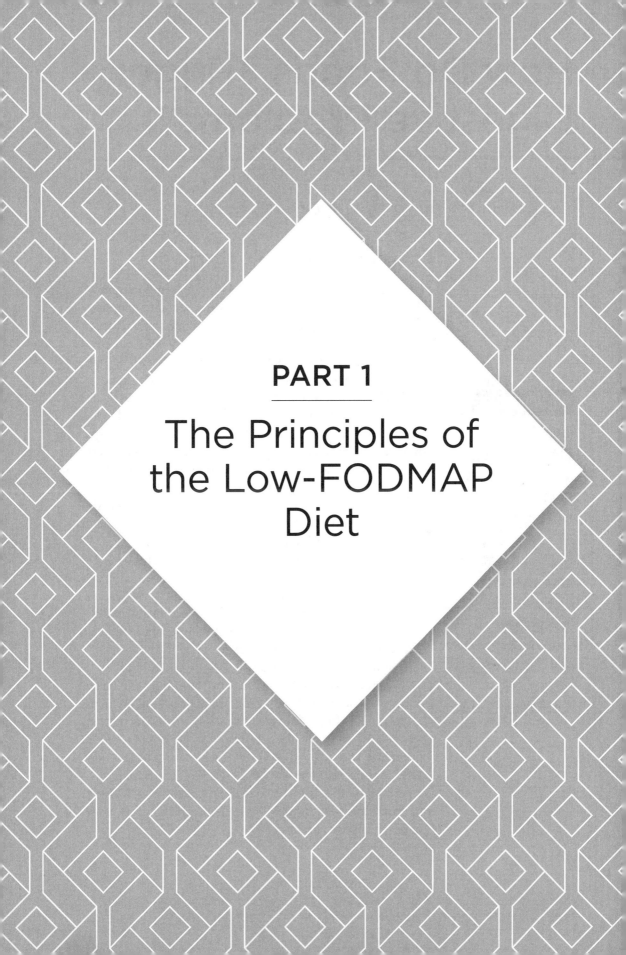

PART 1

The Principles of the Low-FODMAP Diet

How Do Foods Trigger Digestive Problems?

Before discussing the low-FODMAP diet, it's important to understand certain basic principles about how our gastrointestinal (GI) system works.

The Digestive System

The digestive system's main role is to transform foods into energy and useable nutrients for our body, and to eliminate waste. It must also protect our body from anything toxic or harmful to it.

The digestive tract begins at the mouth, where food starts being processed with the help of saliva. Swallowed foods descend to the stomach, thanks to the esophagus's peristaltic movements (rhythmic contractions). In the stomach, food is mixed with hydrochloric acid, which continues the digestive process. The resultant substance, called chyme, then enters the small intestine. This organ is lined with an internal mucous membrane with numerous folds called villi. Villi enable the useful content in digested foods to be absorbed into the bloodstream. It is here that the majority of nutrients and vitamins are absorbed.

The chyme continues digesting and arrives at the large intestine. The undigested part of the chyme is waste. As it migrates along the large intestine, it gradually solidifies as a large part of the water it contains is absorbed by the body. The dried-up waste is then directed to the rectum, at the far end of the large intestine, to be excreted by the anal canal and the anus in the form of stools.

The entire process is controlled by the enteric nervous system (also known as the "second brain"), which functions independently from other nerve centers. The interactions between the brain and the intestine are different in each individual; they depend on several factors, such as emotional state, environment, presence or absence of distractions, experiences and sensitivity to stimuli. Certain people have a malfunctioning enteric nervous system, which makes them more sensitive to stimuli.

DID YOU KNOW?

Helpful Bacteria
The large intestine contains an enormous quantity of bacteria that decompose the carbohydrates that haven't been absorbed within the undigested foods, producing gases and short-chain fatty acids that protect the large intestine's lining.

Food Reactions

The majority of people eat a large variety of foods without encountering the slightest problem. However, for a certain percentage of the population, specific foods or food components can provoke secondary reactions ranging from a slight redness of the skin to a severe allergic response.

Food reactions can be due to an allergy or a food intolerance. Although around one person in three considers themselves allergic to certain foods, in reality the prevalence of allergy is estimated at 2% of the population, while intolerances affect around 20%. The terms "allergy" and "intolerance" are often used interchangeably and inappropriately. In reality, there are two different types of undesirable reactions:

- **Food allergy:** A food allergy is a hypersensitive reaction by the immune system when faced with a dietary protein. An allergen (often a protein within the problematic food) provokes a chain reaction within the immune system, which releases type IgE antibodies. The effects can be immediate or delayed, and are usually localized (for example, sneezing, swelling of the lips, itching and so on). For a small number of people, an allergic reaction can be fatal; this is what's known as anaphylaxis. Food allergies are often hereditary and are usually identified early in life.
- **Food intolerance:** With a food intolerance, the body is incapable of properly digesting a food or food component. An intolerance therefore involves the metabolism, but in no way does it involve the immune system, despite the fact that the symptoms can be similar to those of an allergy (nausea, diarrhea, stomach cramps). Symptoms can appear several hours after the food has been consumed. Whereas allergic persons cannot tolerate even the slightest quantity of an allergen, intolerant persons can often deal with small doses of a problematic food without any symptoms.

A food allergy can be correctly diagnosed by testing for antibodies through blood or skin tests. However, in the case of an intolerance, the signs aren't as easy to detect. In most cases, therefore, we turn to an empirical method — an elimination diet — to discover which foods are problematic. Once the symptoms have disappeared, we carefully reintroduce the potentially responsible foods, one by one, to identify those that cause problems.

DID YOU KNOW?

Food Intolerance Symptoms
Dietary intolerances most often manifest via intestinal discomforts, but also more rarely through other symptoms, such as headaches or fatigue. With regard to the intestinal discomforts, the most frequent is linked to abdominal distension — an increase in the abdomen's size and volume — due to bloating caused by an accumulation of gas in the intestines.

Irritable Bowel Syndrome

Irritable bowel syndrome (IBS), also known as nervous colon, spastic colon and irritable colon, is a functional disorder of the intestine. "Functional" means that it causes problems to the intestine's functioning, even in the absence of physical lesions. In IBS, defecation brings abdominal pain or discomfort, and there may be a change in bowel movement frequency. Bloating, abdominal distension (an increase in the abdomen's size and volume) and intestinal transit disorders are also associated with IBS.

What Are the Symptoms?

The symptoms of IBS are varied, but are always linked to bowel movements and sensitivity — in other words, to the way the brain interprets signals coming from the intestinal nerves. The most common potential symptoms are:

Several factors can contribute to the development of IBS, and they vary from person to person.

- **Severe abdominal pain (cramps):** These vary in length, severity and frequency. Defecation often provides some relief.
- **Diarrhea:** Defecation may be frequent (three times a day or more), with watery or soft stools, and is often accompanied by an urgent need.
- **Constipation:** Alternatively, defecation may be laborious and can occur less than three times a week, with hard, dry stools.

Definition and Diagnosis: The Rome IV Criteria

The symptoms of IBS are varied and, for the moment, no medical test exists to determine whether a patient has it. Therefore, part of the diagnosis process consists of excluding the presence of other known illnesses, which can require blood tests, stool tests, medical imaging and/or food tests. After excluding other causes, the doctor will diagnose IBS if at least two of the following three criteria (the Rome IV criteria) are met:

1. The patient has suffered functional symptoms at least 3 days a month in the last 3 months.
2. The symptoms began at least 6 months ago.
3. The symptoms are lessened after defecating, or they are linked to changes in bowel movements or to changes in their frequency.

- **Other digestive symptoms:** These include alternating between diarrhea and constipation, bloating, gas, nausea, heartburn, mucus in stools and a sensation of incomplete evacuation.
- **Other less frequent problems:** Fatigue and muscle aches (fibromyalgia) are sometimes associated with IBS.

What Causes IBS?

The exact cause of IBS is still unknown, but it is now recognized that affected people's enteric nervous system does not function optimally. In particular:

- **Motility:** The motor function that transports digested foods through the intestines does not operate well, inducing too fast a movement (diarrhea) or too slow a movement (constipation), and thereby provoking spasms and pain.
- **Sensitivity:** The network of nerves surrounding the digestive organs becomes unusually sensitive, which means even a small change in intestinal activity can send pain signals to the brain.

Several factors can contribute to the development of IBS, and they vary from person to person. The most common triggers include:

- Acute gastrointestinal infection
- Traveler's diarrhea
- Food poisoning
- Surgery
- Repeated use of antibiotics or other medications
- Bacterial or hormonal imbalance
- Emotional stress, physical stress or anxiety

How Is IBS Treated?

Although IBS is uncomfortable, it is important to stress that it isn't life-threatening. That said, no curative treatment exists. Available treatments focus instead on eradicating the symptoms — or at least relieving them. These treatments are not universal, as they depend on the symptoms and, especially, individual reactions. Available approaches include changes to lifestyle and diet, medication and complementary medicine.

DID YOU KNOW?

Who Is Affected?
IBS can affect people of all ages, but often manifests in adolescence or early adulthood. It affects women more than men, and there's often a family history. It's the most common gastrointestinal disorder in the world. In North America, the incidence is one of the highest, with 13% to 20% of people suffering from IBS at some point in their lives, of which 40% seek medical care. The others, perhaps experiencing less severe symptoms, treat themselves by changing their lifestyle (for example, by avoiding certain foods and using over-the-counter medications).

Lifestyle Changes

Lifestyle changes can both relieve and prevent symptoms:

- Exercise regularly to activate bowel movements. It isn't necessary to work out intensely; simply walking for 20 to 30 minutes can help.
- Reduce stress. The brain and colon are closely linked. Meditation, yoga and other relaxation techniques can help those suffering from IBS to effectively manage their stress.
- Get enough rest. Lack of sleep and tiredness aggravate symptoms.
- Avoid behaviors that can promote flatulence, namely anything that can cause air to be swallowed into the digestive system (chewing gum, eating quickly, etc.).

Meditation, yoga and other relaxation techniques can help those suffering from IBS to effectively manage their stress.

Diet Changes

In general, people who suffer from IBS already know that certain foods trigger their symptoms, but it can be difficult to recognize and adequately avoid or limit these foods. Until very recently, the following dietary precautions were recommended:

- Avoid fast food.
- Ensure adequate intake of dietary fiber.
- Reduce consumption of "gas-forming" foods, such as broccoli, cauliflower and legumes.
- Eat slowly and at regular intervals.
- Avoid eating meals that are too large or too fatty.
- Avoid drinking too much fluid during a meal.
- Limit consumption of alcohol, coffee and fizzy drinks.

The FODMAP approach is now added to these recommendations. We will explore later, in more detail, the type of dietary changes needed to obtain more effective symptom relief.

Medication

To this day, no medication has been demonstrated to be effective in the treatment of IBS. Nonetheless, some medications effectively treat the symptoms, especially those related to cramps, diarrhea and constipation. Antispasmodics (Dicetel, Modulon), antacids (Nexium, Prevacid, Pantoloc, Zantac), antidiarrheals (Imodium, Questran, Lomotil) and laxatives (Metamucil, lactulose) are often prescribed to control the symptoms associated with IBS.

Complementary Approaches

- **Yoga and hypnotherapy:** Many people suffering from IBS experience real benefits from practicing yoga or attending hypnosis sessions, as these techniques help to reduce anxiety and control stress. It is not yet fully understood how these practices work, but there is plenty of evidence demonstrating their benefits.
- **Probiotics:** Probiotics can also help reduce IBS symptoms. Probiotics are living bacteria that, when consumed regularly and in sufficient quantities, have a potentially beneficial effect on health. Indeed, the intestinal flora of IBS sufferers is different from that of healthy persons. In general, people with IBS have a larger amount of undesirable bacteria and a smaller amount of beneficial bacteria. Research in the field of probiotics is promising and is developing rapidly; however, at this point the results are inconsistent due to a lack of study uniformity.
- **Natural health products:** Among natural health products, peppermint essential oil in tablet form may be effective thanks to its antispasmodic action.

> **DID YOU KNOW?**
> **Acupuncture for IBS**
> Some people turn to acupuncture to reduce their abdominal aches. However, there aren't enough conclusive scientific studies to confirm the effectiveness of this practice on IBS.

IBS Should Not Be Confused With:

Inflammatory Bowel Disease (IBD)

IBS is sometimes confused with IBD, but unlike IBD, IBS does not include structural damage to the intestine. "Inflammatory bowel disease" is a term that refers primarily to two diseases of the intestines: Crohn's disease (which can affect any part of the digestive tract, from the mouth to the anus) and ulcerative colitis (which affects only a limited segment of the rectum and the colon). The cause of these illnesses is not known. Treatments are focused around inflammation control and preventing reoccurrences. Persons suffering from IBD can also have IBS and, depending on their specific symptoms, can benefit from a reduction of certain FODMAPs.

Around one in three people with celiac disease also suffers from IBS.

Celiac Disease

Celiac disease is a chronic autoimmune disease affecting the small intestine. In genetically predisposed individuals, exposure to gluten, even in tiny amounts, causes inflammation that damages the intestinal villi (structures resembling small fingers) that line the intestinal walls. As a result, the damaged intestine becomes unable to adequately absorb nutrients.

Celiac disease is classified as an autoimmune disease because the body damages its own tissues. The only treatment is a strict gluten-free diet for life. With the avoidance of gluten, the intestine can heal and the risk of developing serious complications is diminished.

Individuals suffering from celiac disease sometimes experience symptoms similar to those of IBS, and they can also benefit from a gluten-free, low-FODMAP diet. Indeed, around one in three people with celiac disease also suffers from IBS. Moreover, in the months following a celiac disease diagnosis, a transitional lactose intolerance is often observed, which for certain patients can persist for a long time.

DID YOU KNOW?

Prevalence of SIBO
Between 4% and 18% of healthy people have SIBO. This percentage is up to four times higher for those who suffer from IBS, mainly people with IBS-D (IBS principally with diarrhea). People who suffer from autoimmune diseases, like celiac disease, also appear to experience a higher prevalence of SIBO than the general population.

Small Intestinal Bacterial Overgrowth and IBS

Small intestinal bacterial overgrowth (SIBO) is characterized by an excessive proliferation of bacteria in the small intestine. Normally, the majority of the body's bacteria are found in the large intestine, or colon. However, certain conditions or illnesses can cause bacteria in the colon to migrate up the digestive system toward the small intestine. This can cause digestive symptoms including diarrhea, bloating, wind, abdominal cramps, nausea, dyspepsia, constipation and even fatigue. These nonspecific symptoms make diagnosing SIBO far from straightforward, especially because they resemble the symptoms of other gastrointestinal conditions, such as IBS.

It's important to note that SIBO isn't an illness in itself. Rather, it is a symptom of or the result of an underlying condition. The development of SIBO is associated with several illnesses, including scleroderma, exocrine pancreatic insufficiency, chronic pancreatitis, diverticulitis, diabetes, small intestine inflammation, inflammatory bowel diseases, celiac disease, irritable bowel syndrome, Parkinson's disease, liver disease and arthritis.

Causes of SIBO

Small intestinal bacterial overgrowth is, in most cases, the result of an issue in one of these categories:

- **Motility troubles:** A reduction in the intestine's peristaltic movements creates the perfect environment for bacterial proliferation. Motility troubles are associated with certain illnesses (such as diabetes) and certain medications (such as narcotics). Many people also develop motility issues as they age.
- **Intestinal pH balance:** Certain medications, such as proton pump inhibitors (PPIs), can influence the digestive system's pH balance, which can weaken the small intestine's antibacterial defense, encouraging SIBO to develop.
- **Structural anomalies:** Diverticulitis, tumors or strictures in the small intestine can also encourage the proliferation of bacteria.

SIBO Treatment

There are usually three stages to SIBO treatment. The first stage focuses on inducing remission (stopping the symptoms). To achieve this, antibiotics are usually prescribed to eliminate the bacteria in the small intestine.

The second stage aims to prolong the remission period as long as possible. Unfortunately, SIBO is a condition that tends to come back after a few years. There are several ways to lengthen periods of remission, including prokinetic medications (medicines that promote intestinal movements). Regular intestinal movements create an environment that is less favorable for bacteria to multiply. In healthy people, peristaltic movements in the small intestine are one of the reasons why we don't tend to find many bacteria there. Diet can also play a role in lengthening the periods of remission. A low-FODMAP diet, for example, contains few foods that ferment in the digestive system, and researchers believe that the risk of bacterial proliferation may diminish when gut fermentation is reduced.

The third stage is to treat, if possible, the cause of bacterial overgrowth. As discussed above, the causes are numerous and varied. You'll need to work together with your health-care team to identify the cause and treat it as best as possible.

DID YOU KNOW?

Elemental Diet
A recent scientific discovery has demonstrated that an elemental diet (in liquid form) could be a potential treatment for SIBO. These drinks may be better digested than regular food because the nutritional elements (proteins, carbohydrates and hydrolyzed fats) are digested and absorbed earlier in the digestive system. Further studies are necessary before this type of diet can be recommended, because these drinks are expensive and not very palatable.

The Low-FODMAP Diet

In general, those dealing with IBS already know that certain foods trigger their symptoms. They are therefore receptive to a dietary approach that reduces these symptoms. The low-FODMAP diet has been scientifically proven to be effective in eliminating or considerably reducing IBS symptoms, in both the short term and the long term.

What Does FODMAP Stand For?

FODMAPs are specific carbohydrates (sugars) that are difficult for humans to digest, so they arrive almost intact at the large intestine, where they feed the local bacteria. The acronym stands for fermentable oligosaccharides, disaccharides, monosaccharides and polyols. Let's take a closer look at what these individual words mean:

- **Fermentable:** When carbohydrates are not completely digested in the small intestine, they ferment in the colon instead.
- **Oligosaccharides:** An oligosaccharide is a carbohydrate in which three to ten simple sugars are linked together. In particular, the combination of fructans and galacto-oligosaccharides (GOS) creates fermentable short-chain carbohydrates that the human body cannot digest; these are found mainly in certain vegetables, legumes and grains.
- **Disaccharides:** A disaccharide is a carbohydrate formed from two simple sugars. The combination of galactose and glucose creates lactose, a fermentable short-chain carbohydrate that is present in milk and dairy products. Lactose is the only disaccharide that is part of the FODMAP group.
- **Monosaccharides:** These carbohydrates are made up of a single sugar. Fructose, the only monosaccharide that is part of the FODMAP group, is most commonly found in certain fruits and sweeteners.
- **Polyols:** Also called sugar alcohols, polyols such as sorbitol, mannitol, maltitol, xylitol, polydextrose and isomalt are found mainly in reduced-sugar confectionary.

Why Do FODMAPs Cause IBS Symptoms?

"Saccharide" means sugar: a monosaccharide contains one sugar, a disaccharide contains two, and an oligosaccharide contains "a few" (*oligo*, in Greek), meaning anywhere from three to ten. A polyol is a glycol, or sugar alcohol. All FODMAPs behave similarly in the intestine:

1. FODMAPs are not absorbed completely by the small intestine. We all differ in our capacity to digest and absorb FODMAPs. For some people, the absorption of fructose and polyols is extremely slow. Others are lactose-intolerant because they do not produce enough lactase, the enzyme that breaks down lactose. As for fructans and GOS, these are sugars the human body is unable to digest.
2. FODMAPs are small molecules normally consumed in large quantities through food. When they arrive in the intestine, they create an influx of water by osmosis, which can cause diarrhea in certain people.
3. FODMAPs, like fibers, feed the bacteria present in the colon. The colon contains billions of bacteria, which, while decomposing FODMAPs, quickly produce gases, of which some are beneficial. Because FODMAPs are made up of short-chain molecules, they ferment much more quickly than fibers, which are made up of long-chain molecules.

Several types of FODMAPs are typically consumed in a meal, leading to a cumulative effect on the intestine. That's why we need to consider all of them when modifying our diet.

> We all differ in our capacity to digest and absorb FODMAPs.

Get Help from a Registered Dietitian

The FODMAP approach is designed to be applied with the help of a specialized registered dietitian. Although this book is a very useful tool to help you put the low-FODMAP diet into practice, we recommend that you consult a dietitian who can tailor the approach to your individual needs, especially if you have other health issues in addition to IBS. By analyzing your current dietary habits, the dietitian will be able to pinpoint the main foods that are responsible for your problems and suggest substitutes. He or she will also ensure that you have no deficiencies, and will answer any questions you may have regarding the FODMAP approach.

Where Are FODMAPs Found?

The quantity and type of FODMAPs we are exposed to varies depending on our culinary traditions and the time of year. For example, Indian and Mexican cuisines, which include many legumes, contain large quantities of GOS. During the summer, when stone fruits such as peaches, apricots and prunes fill our markets, we are more exposed to sorbitol.

Oligosaccharides: The Problem with Vegetables, Legumes and Certain Grains

The oligosaccharides are mainly fructans — fructo-oligosaccharides (FOS) and inulins — and galacto-oligosaccharides (GOS).

Fructans

Fructans are made up of fructose molecules with a glucose molecule at the end of the chain. The main sources of fructans are wheat products and vegetables such as onions and garlic. No one digests fructans properly, and they trigger gas in everyone. However, for those suffering from IBS, these gases are painful. Fructans are considered the principal FODMAP, as they're present in a large quantity of common and widely consumed foods.

A food is considered problematic for IBS sufferers when a portion contains more than 0.2 grams of fructan for cereal-based products, or 0.3 grams for other foods.

> No one digests fructans properly, and they trigger gas in everyone.

Where Fructans Are Found

	HIGH-FRUCTAN FOODS	MODERATE-FRUCTAN FOODS	LOW-FRUCTAN FOODS
Vegetables*	artichokes, asparagus, garlic, Jerusalem artichokes, leeks, onions (all), shallots	beets, broccoli, Brussels sprouts, butternut squash, corn, fennel, peas, savoy cabbage, snow peas	alfalfa sprouts, avocados, bamboo shoots, bell peppers (all colors), bok choy, carrots, cauliflower, celery, Chinese cabbage, chives, cucumbers, eggplant, escarole, gingerroot, green beans, lettuces (all), mushrooms (all), olives, parsnips, potatoes, pumpkin, rutabaga, spinach, squash (all except butternut), sweet potatoes, Swiss chard, tomatoes, turnips, water chestnuts, watercress, zucchini
Fruits*	nectarines, persimmons, watermelon, white peaches	grapefruit, pomegranates	all other fruits
Grains	barley, rye products (bread, flour, pasta), wheat and Kamut products (bread, cereals, cookies, couscous, flour, pasta)		amaranth, buckwheat, corn (meal and starch), millet, oats, quinoa, rice, sorghum, tapioca, teff
Legumes	beans (all), black-eyed peas, soybeans, split peas	canned chickpeas (rinsed), canned lentils (rinsed), peanuts, peanut butter	tempeh, tofu
Nuts and seeds	cashews, pistachios	almonds, Brazil nuts, chia seeds, flax seeds, green pumpkin seeds (pepitas), hazelnuts, pine nuts, sesame seeds, sunflower seeds, walnuts, butters from permitted nuts and seeds	
Beverages	chicory-based coffee substitutes	rice beverage	coffee, herbal tea, tea
Fiber supplements	fructo-oligosaccharides, inulin, wheat bran	chia seeds, flax seeds	oat bran, psyllium, rice bran

Source: Monash University Low FODMAP Diet app and other databases. Visit www.soscuisine.com/77880569 to view an updated version of this table.

* When it comes to fruits and vegetables, the quantity of FODMAPs depends on the season, the variety and their degree of maturity. The information in this table should serve as a guide; you will need to establish your own level of tolerance.

Galacto-oligosaccharides

Galacto-oligosaccharides (GOS) are made up of galactose molecules linked together by a fructose molecule and a glucose molecule. They are most commonly found in dried legumes, such as beans, lentils and chickpeas. As with fructans, humans do not properly digest GOS, and people with IBS often need to avoid them. A food is considered problematic when a portion contains more than 0.2 grams of GOS. However, some people can tolerate $\frac{1}{4}$ cup (60 mL) of well-rinsed canned lentils or chickpeas. Indeed, canned legumes are easier to digest than dried ones you cook yourself. This is because GOS contained in lentils and chickpeas are water-soluble and pass into the can's brine. It is therefore important to remember to rinse and drain the legumes properly before consuming them.

> As with fructans, humans do not properly digest GOS, and people with IBS often need to avoid them.

Where GOS Are Found

HIGH-GOS LEGUMES	MODERATE-GOS LEGUMES
beans (all), black-eyed peas, dried chickpeas, dried lentils, soybeans, split peas	canned chickpeas (rinsed), canned lentils (rinsed)

Source: Monash University Low FODMAP Diet app and other databases. Visit www.soscuisine.com/77880569 to view an updated version of this table.

Disaccharides: The Problem with Dairy Products

Among disaccharides, only lactose, or milk sugar, is part of the FODMAP group.

Lactose

Lactose is a sugar present in all animal-derived milks (cow's, sheep's and goat's). The enzyme lactase, present in the human small intestine, decomposes lactose into two simple digestible sugars, glucose and galactose. People who are lactose-intolerant produce insufficient quantities of lactase, so any ingested lactose makes it way almost whole to the colon, where it will be fermented by bacteria and could provoke uncomfortable symptoms. It is therefore important to reduce the quantity of lactose consumed in the elimination phase of the low-FODMAP diet. Note that this does not mean completely avoiding all dairy products, as the amount of lactose present in some products (such as butter and certain cheeses) is negligible. Most people who are lactose-intolerant can tolerate 4 grams per portion without problems. You'll need to establish your own level of tolerance.

Where Lactose Is Found

FOODS	LACTOSE (g)
cow's, goat's and sheep's milk (1 cup/250 mL)	12–16
evaporated milk (½ cup/125 mL)	13
yogurt (¾ cup/175 mL)	6
cheesecake (1 small slice)	6
ice cream (2 scoops/125 mL)	4
ricotta cheese (¼ cup/60 mL)	2
cream cheese (1 tbsp/15 mL)	1
lactose-free milk (1 cup/250 mL)	less than 1
sour cream (1 tbsp/15 mL)	0.5
cream (1 tbsp/15 mL)	0.4
butter (1 tbsp/15 mL)	0.1
hard/aged cheeses, such as Parmesan (1½ oz/50 g)	trace
lactose-free ice cream (2 scoops/125 mL)	trace
lactose-free yogurt (¾ cup/175 mL)	trace

Source: Canadian Nutrient File and other databases.

Monosaccharides: The Problem with Fruits

Among monosaccharides, only fructose is part of the FODMAP group.

Fructose

Fructose is found in abundance in fruits, honey and high-fructose corn syrup, used by the food industry. It is also found in certain vegetables. In order to be well absorbed, fructose must be combined with glucose. When there is more fructose than glucose, absorption is slower and incomplete, and the excess fructose triggers symptoms for those with IBS. This doesn't mean all fruits must be eliminated, but simply that those containing excess fructose need to be avoided. A food is considered problematic when a normal portion (for example an apple) contains 0.2 grams more fructose than glucose.

What's more, since the total amount of sugars accumulates in the intestine, it's important not to consume too much fruit in the same meal, even when you limit yourself to fruits that contain less fructose than glucose. Leave at least 2 or 3 hours between eating (meals or snacks), and don't consume more than one portion of fruit — around $1/2$ cup (125 mL) or a fruit the size of a medium orange.

> In order to be well absorbed, fructose must be combined with glucose.

Where Fructose Is Found

	FOODS WITH EXCESS FREE FRUCTOSE	LOW-FRUCTOSE AND BALANCED-FRUCTOSE FOODS
Fruits*	apples (all), boysenberries, cherries, dried fruits, figs, fruit juices, mangos, pears (all), tamarillos, watermelon	apricots, avocados, bananas, blackberries, blueberries, cantaloupe, clementines, cranberries, grapefruit, grapes, honeydew melon, kiwifruit, lemons, limes, nectarines, oranges, papayas, passion fruit, peaches, pineapples, plums (all), raspberries, rhubarb, strawberries, tangerines
Vegetables*	artichokes, asparagus, Jerusalem artichokes, sugar snap peas	all other vegetables
Sweeteners	agave nectar, fructose, high-fructose corn syrup, honey, molasses	glucose, jams,** maple syrup, rice syrup, sucrose (table sugar, powdered/icing sugar, brown sugar, etc.)

Source: Monash University Low FODMAP Diet app and other databases. Visit www.soscuisine.com/77880569 to view an updated version of this table.

∗ When it comes to fruits and vegetables, the quantity of FODMAPs depends on the season, the variety and their degree of maturity. The information in this table should serve as a guide; you will need to establish your own level of tolerance.

∗∗ Be careful with 100% fruit jams, as they are often sweetened with fruit juice.

Polyols: The Problem with Sugar Alcohols and Some Fruits and Vegetables

Polyols are sugar alcohols, which is why their names end in "-ol." The main polyols are sorbitol, mannitol and xylitol. These sugars are naturally present in certain fruits and vegetables, but it is their role as artificial sweeteners in sugar-free candy that causes a problem. Their presence is easy to detect if the label carries a warning along the lines of: "Excessive consumption can lead to laxative effects." A food is considered problematic when a portion contains more than 0.5 grams of polyols.

If you suffer from intestinal discomfort, the first thing to do, and the easiest, is to stop chewing gum and eating sugar-free sweets, because even very small quantities can trigger digestive troubles 30 minutes to 3 hours after ingestion.

Where Polyols Are Found

	HIGH-POLYOL FOODS	MODERATE-POLYOL FOODS	LOW-POLYOL FOODS
Fruits*	apples (all), apricots, avocados, blackberries, cherries, nectarines, peaches (all), pears (all), plums (all), prunes, watermelon	lychees	bananas, blueberries, cantaloupe, carambola, cranberries, grapefruit, grapes, honeydew melon, kiwifruit, lemons, limes, mangos, oranges, papayas, passion fruit, pineapples, raspberries, rhubarb, strawberries, tangerines
Vegetables*	butternut squash, cauliflower, mushrooms (all), snow peas	celery, sweet potatoes	all other vegetables
Sweeteners	*foods sweetened with:* isomalt, maltitol, mannitol, polydextrose, sorbitol, xylitol		*foods sweetened with:* aspartame, glucose, saccharin, stevia, sucrose
Beverages		coconut water	

Source: Monash University Low FODMAP Diet app and other databases. Visit www.soscuisine.com/77880569 to view an updated version of this table.

*When it comes to fruits and vegetables, the quantity of FODMAPs depends on the season, the variety and their degree of maturity. The information in this table should serve as a guide; you will need to establish your own level of tolerance.

How to Benefit from the Low-FODMAP Diet

The FODMAP approach offers a double benefit: during the first phase, it helps to rapidly and considerably reduce symptoms in most people dealing with IBS; during the second phase, it helps to make the most of the benefits of a varied diet by precisely identifying problem foods, which are the only ones that need to be avoided or limited.

Following a low-FODMAP diet often means important changes in the way you nourish yourself. Ideally, to obtain the best possible results, it is best to consult a registered dietitian with experience in this approach; he or she will help to adapt it to your specific needs and will be able to answer all your questions.

The more rigorously you follow the program, without exceptions, the more quickly you will see results.

DID YOU KNOW?

Test for Celiac Disease First

Before applying the FODMAP approach, it's essential to verify whether you suffer from celiac disease. Indeed, removing gluten from the diet can prevent celiac disease from being correctly diagnosed.

Phase 1: Elimination of FODMAPs

The first phase of the low-FODMAP diet — complete elimination of FODMAPs — lasts between 2 and 6 weeks, depending on the person. The more rigorously you follow the program, without exceptions, the more quickly you will see results. You might notice improvements in the first week, but it's important to achieve stable intestinal well-being before moving on to the second phase, when problematic foods are identified.

To make your task easier, you can follow the detailed meal plans, with corresponding recipes, found in part 2 of this book. These meal plans are designed to help you eliminate FODMAPs from your diet while ensuring that you avoid developing nutritional deficiencies. If you follow them strictly, you should quickly observe a substantial improvement in your symptoms.

You can also subscribe online at www.soscuisine.com/FODMAP to receive low-FODMAP meal plans personalized to your preferences. These also come with recipes and a complete grocery list.

If you wish to design your own meal plans and adapt your own recipes, be sure to eliminate all types of FODMAPs: fructans, GOS, lactose, fructose in excess of glucose, and polyols. During the elimination phase, it is preferable to use simple ingredients and avoid processed foods that contain several ingredients (for example, prepared sauces made with garlic or onions). For the same reason, avoid restaurants during the elimination phase.

The tables on pages 31–33 will help you create your meal plans by telling you which foods are allowed during the elimination phase (low-FODMAP foods) and which foods to avoid (high-FODMAP foods). Because it's the combined effect of all the FODMAPs that triggers symptoms, pay attention to your entire diet, including foods that contain only a moderate amount of FODMAPs.

Allowed Foods

Fruits (1 piece, unless otherwise indicated)

banana (small: 5 oz/150 g, or ½ large)	honeydew melon (½ cup/125 mL chopped)
berries (½ cup/125 mL): blueberries, cranberries, raspberries, strawberries	kiwifruit
	lychees (5)
cantaloupe (½ cup/125 mL chopped)	papaya (½ cup/125 mL chopped)
citrus fruits: clementines (2), grapefruit (½ fruit: 4 oz/125 g), lemon, lime, mandarin orange, orange, tangerine	passionfruit (2)
	pineapple (½ cup/125 mL chopped canned or fresh)
dragon fruit (½ cup/125 mL chopped)	rhubarb (½ cup/125 mL chopped)
grapes (¾ cup/175 mL)	

Vegetables and herbs

bamboo shoots	lettuces (all)
bell peppers (all colors)	okra (60 g)
bok choy	parsnips
broccoli (½ cup/125 mL chopped or 60 g)	peas (20 g)
Brussels sprouts (2)	potatoes
carrots	radishes
celeriac	rutabaga
celery (½ stalk/20 g)	savoy cabbage (½ cup/125 mL or 40 g)
Chinese cabbage (½ cup/125 mL or 40 g)	soybean sprouts
corn (¼ cup/60 mL or 30 g)	spinach
cucumber	squash (all except butternut)
eggplant	sweet potato (⅓ cup/75 mL chopped or 70 g)
endive	
fennel (½ cup/125 mL chopped or 45 g)	Swiss chard
gingerroot	tomatoes
green beans	turnips
hearts of palm	water chestnuts
herbs (all)	zucchini
kale	

Sweeteners (in moderation)

brown rice syrup	maple syrup
brown sugar	sugar
dark chocolate	

Allowed Foods (*continued*)

Seasonings, spices and fats

butter	olives
ketchup (in moderation)	shortenings
margarine	soy sauce
mayonnaise	spices
mustard	tomato paste (100% tomato)
oils	vinegar

Beverages

beer (12 oz/341 mL)	tea (except chai or oolong)
coconut water (3½ oz/100 mL)	water
coffee (in moderation)	wine (4 oz/125 mL; no sweet wines)
herbal tea (except chamomile, dandelion or fennel)	

Dairy products and alternatives

almond milk	hemp milk
cheeses (1 oz/28 g): blue, Brie, Camembert, Cheddar, cream cheese (2 tbsp/30 mL plain), Edam, Emmental, feta, Gorgonzola, Gouda, Gruyère, Haloumi, Havarti, mozzarella, Parmesan, pecorino, raclette, Stilton, Swiss	lactose-free ice cream
	lactose-free milk
	lactose-free yogurt
	rice milk (7 oz/200 mL)
coconut milk (canned)	soy milk (made exclusively from soy protein, not from whole soybeans)

Protein sources

canned chickpeas, well rinsed (¼ cup/60 mL)	peanuts (2 tbsp/30 mL)
canned lentils, well rinsed (¼ cup/60 mL)	peanut butter and butters made from other permitted nuts and seeds
eggs	seeds (2 tbsp/30 mL): chia seeds, flax seeds, green pumpkin seeds (pepitas), sesame seeds, sunflower seeds
fish and shellfish (all, unprocessed)	
meat and poultry (all, unprocessed)	seitan
nuts (2 tbsp/30 mL unless otherwise indicated): almonds (10), Brazil nuts, hazelnuts (10), macadamia nuts, pecans, pine nuts, walnuts	tempeh
	tofu

Grains and grain products (flours, breads, cereals, crackers and pasta made from these grains)

amaranth	rice
buckwheat	sorghum
corn	tapioca
millet	teff
oats	wild rice
quinoa	

Source: Monash University Low-FODMAP Diet app and other databases. Visit www.soscuisine.com/77880569 to view an updated version of this table.

Foods to Avoid

Fruits

apples	figs	plums
apricots	mangos	prunes
avocados	nectarines	tamarillos
blackberries	peaches	watermelon
cherries	pears	dried fruits
dates	persimmons	fruit juices

Vegetables

artichokes	cauliflower	mushrooms
asparagus	garlic	onions (all)
beets	Jerusalem artichokes	snow peas
butternut squash	leeks	sugar snap peas

Grains and grain products

barley	rye products: bread, flour	wheat and Kamut products: bread, cookies, couscous, flour, pasta
breakfast cereals made from barley, rye or wheat		

Meat, poultry, fish and egg dishes made from high-FODMAP ingredients

sausages	sauces	stocks and broths

Legumes

beans (all)	dried lentils	split peas
dried chickpeas	soybeans	

Nuts

cashews	pistachios

Dairy products and alternatives

condensed milk	milk (cow's, goat's, sheep's)	soy products (milk, yogurt) made from whole soybeans
evaporated milk	soft cheeses: cottage cheese, flavored cream cheese, mascarpone, quark, ricotta	yogurt
ice cream		
kefir		

Sweeteners

agave nectar	honey	molasses

Beverages

black currant liqueur	coolers	sweet wines: Marsala, Muscat, port, Sauternes, vermouth
chicory-based coffee substitutes	fruit juices	
cider	Pernod	
	rum	

Source: Monash University Low-FODMAP Diet app and other databases. Visit www.soscuisine.com/77880569 to view an updated version of this table.

High-FODMAP Food Alternatives

HIGH-FODMAP FOODS TO AVOID	PERMITTED FOODS (WHEN CONSUMED IN SPECIFIED OR NORMALLY CONSUMED QUANTITIES)
Grain products	
bread made from wheat (white or whole wheat) or rye	100% spelt sourdough bread, corn tortillas (100%), gluten-free bread*
barley, bulgur, couscous, egg noodles, farro, udon noodles, wheat or rye pasta	amaranth, corn, gluten-free pasta,* millet, polenta, quinoa, rice (all), rice noodles, 100% buckwheat soba noodles
most breakfast cereals	corn cereals, gluten-free breakfast cereals,* oatmeal, puffed rice, quinoa flakes
cakes, pastries and other bakery products made from wheat flour	flourless cakes, gluten-free bakery products*
flours made from chickpeas, lentils, peas, rye, soy or wheat, semolina, wheat bran, wheat germ	flours made from amaranth, buckwheat, millet, oats, quinoa, rice, sorghum, tapioca or teff, cornmeal, corn starch
Dairy products	
fresh and soft cheeses	cream cheese (plain, 2 tbsp/30 mL), goat cheese (¼ cup/60 mL), hard/aged cheeses (1 oz/28 g): blue, Brie, Camembert, Cheddar, Edam, Emmental, feta, Gorgonzola, Gouda, Gruyère, Haloumi, Havarti, mozzarella, Parmesan, pecorino, raclette, Stilton, Swiss
cow's, goat's and sheep's milk, evaporated milk, yogurt	butter, cream (2 tbsp/30 mL), sour cream (¼ cup/60 mL), almond milk, hemp milk, rice milk (7 oz/200 mL), soy milk (made exclusively from soy protein, not from whole soybeans), lactose-free ice cream, lactose-free milk, lactose-free yogurt
Meats and substitutes	
sausages	eggs, fish and shellfish, meat and poultry (unprocessed and unseasoned), seitan, tempeh, tofu
ready-to-use chicken or beef broth	homemade chicken or beef stock made from low-FODMAP ingredients
Nuts and seeds	
cashews, pistachios	*2 tbsp (30 mL) of the following foods, unless otherwise indicated:* almonds (10), Brazil nuts (10), chia seeds, flax seeds, green pumpkin seeds (pepitas), hazelnuts (10), peanuts, pine nuts (1 tbsp/15 mL), sesame seeds, sunflower seeds, walnuts (10), butters made from peanuts or permitted nuts and seeds

HIGH-FODMAP FOODS TO AVOID	PERMITTED FOODS (WHEN CONSUMED IN SPECIFIED OR NORMALLY CONSUMED QUANTITIES)
Legumes	
beans (all), dried chickpeas, dried lentils, soybeans, split peas	canned chickpeas or lentils, well rinsed (¼ cup/60 mL), tempeh, tofu
Vegetables	
artichokes, asparagus, beets, butternut squash, cauliflower, garlic, Jerusalem artichokes, leeks, mushrooms, onions (all), shallots, snow peas, sugar snap peas	alfalfa sprouts, bamboo shoots, bell peppers (all), bok choy, broccoli (½ cup/125 mL chopped), Brussels sprouts (2), carrots, celery (½ stalk), Chinese cabbage (½ cup/125 mL), collard greens, corn (¼ cup/60 mL), cucumber, eggplant, fennel (½ cup/125 mL chopped), gingerroot, green and wax beans, hearts of palm, herbs (all), lettuces (all), okra (60 g), parsnips, peas (20 g), potatoes, radishes, rutabaga, savoy cabbage (½ cup/125 mL), soybean sprouts, spinach, squash (all except butternut), sweet potato (⅓ cup/75 mL), Swiss chard, tomatoes, turnips, water chestnuts, watercress, zucchini
ready-to-use vegetable stock	homemade vegetable stock made from low-FODMAP ingredients
Fruits	
apples, apricots, avocados, blackberries, cherries, dates, dried fruits, figs, mangos, nectarines, peaches, pears, persimmons, plums, prunes, tamarillos, watermelon, fruit juice	*½ cup (125 mL) of the following foods, unless otherwise indicated:* banana (small or ½ large), blueberries, cantaloupe, carambola, clementines, cranberries, dragon fruit, grapes, grapefruit (½ fruit), guava, honeydew melon, kiwifruit, lemons, limes, lychees (5), mandarin oranges, oranges, papayas, passion fruit, pineapple (fresh or canned), pomegranate seeds (¼ cup/60 mL), prickly pears, raspberries, rhubarb, strawberries, tangerines
Sweeteners	
isomalt, maltitol, mannitol, polydextrose, sorbitol, xylitol	aspartame, glucose, saccharin, stevia, sucrose
agave nectar, fructose, fruit juice concentrate, high-fructose corn syrup, honey, molasses	brown sugar, glucose, granulated (white) sugar, jam (made from low-FODMAP fruits and sweetened with sucrose), maple syrup, powdered (icing) sugar, rice syrup

High-FODMAP Food Alternatives (*continued*)

HIGH-FODMAP FOODS TO AVOID	PERMITTED FOODS (WHEN CONSUMED IN SPECIFIED OR NORMALLY CONSUMED QUANTITIES)
Beverages	
chai tea, chamomile tea, chicory-based coffee substitutes, dandelion tea, fennel tea, fruit juice, oolong tea	coconut water (3½ oz/100 mL), coffee (in moderation), herbal tea (except chamomile, dandelion, fennel), orange or grapefruit juice (½ cup/125 mL), tea (except chai and oolong), water
black currant liqueur, cider, coolers, Pernod, rum, sweet wines (Marsala, Muscat, port, Sauternes, vermouth)	beer (12 oz/341 mL) and wine (4 oz/125 mL)
Fats	
nil	butter, ghee, lard, margarine, vegetable oils
Other	
ready-made seasonings, sauces and vinaigrettes	baking powder, baking soda, dried tomatoes (4), ketchup (4 tsp/20 mL), mayonnaise, mustard, salt, soy sauce, spices, tomato paste (100% tomato), vinegar
Fiber supplements	
fructo-oligosaccharides, inulin, wheat bran	chia and flax seeds (2 tbsp/30 mL), oat bran, psyllium, rice bran

Source: Monash University Low-FODMAP Diet app and other databases. Visit www.soscuisine.com/77880569 to view an updated version of this table.

* Gluten-free breads and products are a good alternative, but make sure they do not contain any high-FODMAP ingredients such as fruit juice concentrate, honey, inulin or nut flours.

Soy: Low or High FODMAP?

Understanding foods' FODMAP content isn't always easy. One of the foods that many people are confused about is soy. This confusion is partly due to the fact many different products are derived from soy (soy milk, tofu in all its forms, tempeh, edamame, etc.) and some of them are high in FODMAPS while others are low in FODMAPs! How can you tell the difference? Keep reading.

Soy and its derived products can contain fructans, galacto-oligosaccharides (GOS) or both. Depending on the type of processing the soybean goes through, these FODMAPs are either destroyed or not. What you should remember is that it isn't necessary to remove all soy products from your diet, even during the FODMAP elimination phase. While soybeans are rich in FODMAPs, most soy products contain only small to moderate amounts.

Edamame vs Soybeans

You might think that edamame and soybeans are the same thing. Technically, you're absolutely right. The difference between edamame and soybeans is the bean's level of maturity. Edamame are soybeans that have not yet reached maturity. That's why a small amount of edamame is considered low in FODMAPs — up to 1 cup (250 mL) or $3\frac{1}{2}$ oz (100 g) in the pod, or about $\frac{1}{2}$ cup (125 mL) or $1\frac{1}{2}$ oz (50 g) without the pod. Soybeans, on the other hand, are rich in FODMAPs, whatever the amount.

Fermented Soy Foods

Fermenting soy helps to diminish its FODMAP content. The most common foods made from fermented soybeans are tempeh, miso paste and soy sauce. All three are low in FODMAPs, as long as they're not seasoned with high-FODMAP ingredients, like garlic or onions.

Tempeh is an excellent meat alternative. It cooks like tofu but is tastier. You can find it in the frozen section in most health food shops and some grocery stores.

Soy Milk and Yogurt

Depending how it is processed, soy milk can have a high or low FODMAP content — just to add to the confusion! In fact, it's quite simple. Soy milk is made from either whole soybeans (high FODMAP content) or soy proteins only (low FODMAP content). If you find soy milk made from soy protein, you can use it to replace lactose-free milk or almond milk.

Most soy yogurts are produced from soy milk made from whole soybeans. You should therefore avoid them during the FODMAP elimination phase. Lactose-free yogurts (which can be made at home with low-FODMAP milks) are a better choice during this period.

Tofu

Several types of tofu exist, and their FODMAP content varies. Regular tofu is low in FODMAPs, while silken tofu is high in FODMAPs. To understand why the FODMAP content of these two types differs, you simply need to look at the processing methods. Whether silken or regular, the initial process is the same: soy milk is coagulated. For silken tofu, the process stops there. For regular tofu, however, the mix is pressed to remove the water it contains. It is this removal of water that makes regular tofu low in FODMAPs. The FODMAPs present in the original soy milk leach into the water and are therefore absent (or present in tiny quantities) from the final product.

Soy Protein Supplements

When it comes to soy protein supplements, we cannot tell you whether they are low or high in FODMAPs because there are so many different brands, each using different ingredients. But here's a tip to help you choose a soy protein supplement: look at the Nutrition Facts label. If the product doesn't contain any fiber, the chances are it is low in FODMAPs.

Phase 2: Reintroduction of FODMAPs

FODMAP intolerance isn't an allergy. If one is allergic to tree nuts, for example, the slightest trace of nuts in food can have grave consequences, including anaphylactic shock. As for FODMAPs, they ferment in the intestine and the effect is cumulative. This means that, often, a small amount will pose little or no problem. Each individual must determine his or her own tolerance to the various FODMAPs.

After you have followed phase 1 for long enough to be free of symptoms (between 2 and 6 weeks), you can begin phase 2, in which FODMAP reintroduction tests will take place. It is essential to introduce one FODMAP at a time, to precisely identify the food or foods that cause you problems, as well as the quantity you can tolerate. This process is called a "food challenge."

The rules of the challenge are:

1. Test a single type of FODMAP at a time.
2. Test one FODMAP per week.
3. Choose a food that contains only one type of FODMAP in order to avoid confusion when interpreting the results.
4. Choose the quantity you would habitually consume. If you are worried, start with a smaller amount, then increase it if there are no symptoms.
5. Carry out the test in between meals, after a 2-hour fast and 2 hours before eating anything.
6. Repeat the test once more during the week (or until symptoms appear) to confirm the results.
7. Continue to limit other FODMAPs until the end of that FODMAP's challenge.

Pay attention to your symptoms. If you don't experience any, you can, in the same week, increase the quantity, if it was different from what you usually consume, test another food from the same group or repeat the same test to confirm the results. Two tests per food are needed for a conclusive result. Wait at least 48 hours between tests.

If you experience symptoms (bloating, gas, diarrhea, etc.), you can, in the same week, wait until they subside, then test again, diminishing the quantity by half. Alternatively, you can try another food from the same group to confirm the results.

The order in which you reintroduce FODMAPs is not important. However, it is crucial to ascertain that the food used for the test contains only one type of FODMAP. For example, yellow peaches are a good candidate to check your sorbitol sensitivity, but nectarines and white peaches are not, as they also contain fructans. Is it crucial to test all the families of FODMAP.

Although you can reintroduce FODMAPs in any order, the table below provides an example of how you might go about it. As you can see, an entire week is dedicated to onions, because they have such an important role in cuisines from all cultures that it is very important to establish your individual threshold.

For more information on reintroduction, please visit our IBS/low-FODMAP support group on Facebook. To receive an invitation to join the group, visit www.soscuisine.com/77880569.

Sample Reintroduction Schedule

Week 1	Sorbitol	1 yellow peach, ½ avocado or 8 blackberries
Week 2	Mannitol	5-6 white mushrooms or ½ cup (125 mL) chopped cauliflower
Week 3	Lactose	½ to 1 cup (125 to 250 mL) milk or 7 oz (200 g) yogurt
Week 4	Excess fructose	1 tsp (5 mL) honey or ½ mango
Week 5	Fructans (except onion)	2 slices bread, 1 bagel or 1 garlic clove
Week 6	Fructans (onion)	¼ onion (2½ oz/50 g), cooked
Week 7	GOS	½ cup (125 mL) canned legumes or 1 cup (250 mL) soy milk

Frequently Asked Questions

How long does the first phase of the low-FODMAP diet last?

It all depends on how you react. The goal is to achieve complete intestinal well-being before moving on to the reintroduction phase. Your symptoms could be much improved after 2 weeks even if your troubles date back years. But you mustn't rush into phase 2. In general, we recommend following phase 1 for 4 weeks.

How much fruit is allowed, and at what times of the day?

You can eat fruit during meals or in between meals, as you prefer. During each "food intake" (meal or snack), limit yourself to one portion of allowed fruit (see page 31). If you monitor quantities and leave 2 to 3 hours between each food intake, you shouldn't have any problems.

I'm a vegetarian. What protein foods can I eat?

Following a low-FODMAP diet while avoiding meat is more complicated, as legumes, which are the basis of a vegetarian diet, contain GOS and fructans. It is necessary, therefore, to either eliminate legumes or limit the amount consumed, depending on the type of legume. You can consume without problems around $\frac{1}{4}$ cup (60 mL) of well-rinsed canned lentils or chickpeas, as they are lower in FODMAPs than dried beans cooked at home. You can also eat tofu, tempeh, quinoa, eggs, nuts (except pistachios and cashews) and seeds in limited amounts, hard/aged cheeses (such as Parmesan) and lactose-free milk.

DID YOU KNOW?

Meats and Fish

All meats and all fish are allowed in the low-FODMAP diet, as they don't contain any sugar. However, you must ensure that they are not served with sauces containing FODMAPs (for example, garlic or onions).

I'm a vegan. What sources of plant-based protein can I eat?

You can follow the same advice given to vegetarians (opposite), except that you will obviously avoid the cheeses, eggs and lactose-free milk. On page 64, you will find a complete 7-day vegan meal plan, and in part 3 you will find 53 vegan recipes as well as 29 recipes that can be easily adapted to avoid animal products. If you are concerned about nutrient deficiencies or have any specific needs, you may want to consult a registered dietitian.

....

I have celiac disease. Will the FODMAP approach suit me?

Absolutely. Actually, some celiac disease sufferers also suffer from IBS. Celiacs must apply the FODMAP approach while also taking care to eliminate all traces of gluten. Soy sauce, for example, must be strictly gluten-free for celiacs.

....

I have an inflammatory bowel disease. Will the FODMAP approach suit me?

Absolutely. In fact, some people continue to suffer from IBS-type digestive symptoms even when their inflammatory bowel disease (Crohn's disease or ulcerative colitis) is properly treated. In this case, the FODMAP diet is recommended.

....

I have diabetes. Will the FODMAP approach suit me?

Absolutely. In fact, many of the recommendations in the low-FODMAP diet are similar to those for people with diabetes: eating small, regular meals spaced evenly throughout the day, limiting consumption of processed foods. In the meal plans on pages 58–65, the distribution of carbohydrates throughout the day and the allocation of carbohydrates, proteins and fats in each meal have been designed especially to work well for people with diabetes.

DID YOU KNOW?

Weight Loss
The low-FODMAP diet isn't a weight-loss diet, but if you suffer from bloating, it will help you deflate and regain a flatter tummy. In addition, you may lose weight thanks to consuming fewer processed foods, but this isn't guaranteed.

Diabetes and IBS

Diabetes and IBS are both extremely prevalent in the western world. Although there is no link between the incidence of diabetes and that of IBS, a suitable diet will lead to better management of both conditions. In both cases, special attention should be paid to the amount, the quality and the type of carbohydrates consumed. You might think the solution is to avoid carbohydrates altogether, but unfortunately it is not so simple. Carbohydrates play a crucial role in supplying energy to the brain and the rest of the body. It is important to eat some carbohydrates at every meal — in reasonable amounts, of course.

How do you eat well when you have diabetes and IBS? The tips below will help you follow the low-FODMAP diet while also keeping your diabetes in check.

- **Fruits and vegetables:** Eat at least 2 servings of low-FODMAP fruits and 4 servings of low-FODMAP vegetables per day (see page 31). Go for fresh fruits and vegetables rather than juices or dried fruits. Fresh fruits and vegetables contain more fiber than juices and are also more satisfying. Dried fruits are more concentrated in sugars and can more easily have an effect on blood sugar.
- **Grains:** Choose low-FODMAP breads that are high in fiber and made from whole grains. Gluten-free breads (without wheat, barley or rye) are a good alternative, but make sure they don't contain any high-FODMAP ingredients such as concentrated fruit juice, honey, inulin or nut flours. Enjoy whole-grain products such as brown rice, polenta, oats or quinoa to supplement your meal.
- **Dairy products:** Choose low-fat dairy products and, if necessary, lactose-free or low-lactose products.
- **Meats and alternatives:** Most meats and alternatives are carbohydrate-free and therefore do not pose a problem. Legumes are the only fly in the ointment, so test your personal tolerance to legumes. Canned lentils and chickpeas are considered to be low in FODMAPs, as long as you don't eat more than ¼ cup (60 mL).

If I eliminate several fiber-rich foods, will I suffer from constipation?

When you change your dietary habits, there's always a risk of constipation, but if you follow the menus and recipes in this book, you will consume enough fiber to avoid being constipated. Don't forget to hydrate, and do some physical exercise to facilitate bowel movements.

What should I do if I want to eat something that has yet to be tested for FODMAPs?

It depends. If you have already eaten it a few times without symptoms, then you can continue eating it. If it's a new food to you, it's best to wait until you have completed the elimination phase.

Does cooking affect a food's FODMAP content?

No. The FODMAP content is generally not modified by cooking; however, other processes may alter it. For example, canned beans have a lower FODMAP content than soaked dried legumes. Pickling also seems to reduce the FODMAP content of some high-FODMAP foods, such as garlic, onions and beets. The results of these tests are still preliminary, but it will be interesting to see the outcome of further studies!

Do I really have to avoid onions and garlic?

Onions are one of the foods most responsible for triggering IBS symptoms, as they are rich in fructans and omnipresent in cooking. They must, therefore, be completely avoided during the elimination phase, even in small quantities. It is also necessary to avoid their close relatives, such as leeks, shallots and the white part of green onions. Any premade foods that contain onions, such as ready-to-use broths, soups and ready-made sauces, must also be avoided. When you cook with onions, a large part of their FODMAPs ends up in the rest of the dish. Removing the onion at the end of the cooking process is not enough.

Garlic also contains fructans, but if you can't live without it, there's a simple trick: infuse oil by sautéing a whole clove in the oil for 1 minute. You can then use this flavored oil, but make sure to discard the clove of garlic.

When you cook with onions, a large part of their FODMAPs ends up in the rest of the dish. Removing the onion at the end of the cooking process is not enough.

Is it absolutely necessary to avoid all foods that contain wheat?

Yes, unless they contain mere traces of wheat (as with soy sauce, for example). Of course, if you also suffer from celiac disease, you must also avoid all traces of gluten, and therefore of wheat. Certain gluten-free products can easily replace breads, pastas, etc., but it's important to carefully read the ingredient list to ensure that they do not contain any high-FODMAP foods, such as honey (page 33).

What breads should I choose?

Gluten-free breads are a good choice; just make sure to choose one that has no high-FODMAP ingredients, such as honey or legume flours (see page 33). An alternative is to choose a 100% spelt sourdough bread. The slow rise of sourdough bread allows the bacteria to digest some of the FODMAPs contained in spelt.

Does a low-FODMAP diet mean a gluten-free diet?

No, it isn't the same thing. FODMAPs are carbohydrates, whereas gluten is a protein. Many foods that are fine in a gluten-free diet, such as apples, honey and legumes, are eliminated or restricted in a low-FODMAP diet. However, gluten-free products are often appropriate for people following a low-FODMAP diet.

How do I know what I can eat?

Consult the table on pages 34–36 to understand how to substitute one food for another. Then read the advice in "Making the Low-FODMAP Diet Easier" (page 48), follow the meal plans (pages 57–65) and prepare the many delicious recipes in this book.

What can I snack on?

You have plenty of choices. Here are a few ideas: popcorn; a rice cake with nut butter; gluten-free crispbread with ripened hard cheese; crudités with a low-FODMAP dip (lactose-free yogurt with a touch of lemon juice and Dijon mustard, for example); lactose-free yogurt and berries; or the Cranberry Granola Bars (page 82).

Sourdough Bread: Better for the Gut?

Sourdough bread is made from leaven, a mixture of water and flour in which, over a period of several days, a culture of yeast and lactobacilli (a type of bacteria) develops. (Both the yeast and the bacteria are naturally present in flour and the environment.) This mixture is called a starter. The flour is then fermented by the culture. The fermentation enables the dough to rise during cooking by releasing carbon dioxide. This is the oldest known method for obtaining leavened bread. Unlike regular breads, sourdough breads do not need baker's yeast to rise.

During the preparation of sourdough bread, the long fermentation period enables the yeast and lactobacilli to digest some of the carbohydrates and proteins present in the flour, including fructans and gluten. Thus, sourdough breads can typically be eaten without problem by people who suffer from IBS or non-celiac gluten sensitivity (NCGS).

However, sourdough breads are not all the same. The length of the fermentation period is of paramount importance; it must be long enough to enable the bacteria and yeast to digest the carbohydrates and proteins found in flour. For certain commercial sourdough breads available in supermarkets, the process is shortened and other ingredients are added to give the bread the same flavor without allowing enough time for proper fermentation.

If you're interested, ask your baker about his or her process. The majority of artisanal bakeries offering this type of bread make it the traditional way.

Here are two more good reasons to give sourdough bread a try:

- Its shelf life is longer than that of traditional bread. Indeed, the more acidic nature of sourdough bread slows the development of mold and keeps the bread moist for longer — up to a week or even more.
- As indicated by its name, sourdough bread has a slightly sour or tart flavor that is appreciated by many, especially for toasting. Try a slice of toasted sourdough in the morning or enjoy one alongside a main dish.

In brief, sourdough bread is worth a try regardless of your condition, but especially if you are sensitive to fructans (FODMAP) or have NCGS.

The Worst Things to Say to Someone with IBS

Ask your loved ones, friends and coworkers to read this, to help them better understand your condition and how to be helpful.

1. "It's all in your head."

Although we don't yet know the precise cause of IBS, it is certainly not something that is only in the sufferer's head! IBS is a disorder with many factors that affect several of the body's systems, including, of course, the digestive system, but also the nervous system and microbiota. Several hypotheses are currently being researched. It is possible that IBS may be explained by an altered microbiota, a communication problem within the gut-brain axis or visceral hypersensitivity.

2. "Just relax."

It is true that stress can exacerbate the symptoms related to IBS, but saying "just relax" really doesn't help: such a statement can be more stressful than calming. Instead, suggest a relaxing activity you can do together, such as yoga or meditation, to help the IBS sufferer better manage stress.

3. "You stunk up the bathroom."

The person suffering from IBS already knows this; there's no need to notify the entire household! Embarrassing them might even worsen their symptoms by making them feel more sensitive about their symptoms. Not saying anything won't change your life in any way, but will probably make theirs easier.

4. "Let's eat out."

You may think this is a harmless proposition, but it's best to leave the choice to the person with IBS — or at least consult them. IBS symptoms are aggravated or reduced depending on which foods are eaten. It is therefore important that the IBS sufferer choose a restaurant that offers dishes that suit their needs. Ideally, arrange the outing several days before so they can, if needed, consult the menu in advance or phone the restaurant.

One last little tip for the road: Don't try to keep an eye on everything an IBS sufferer eats. They know themselves well enough to know which foods work for them and which don't. However, if you want to familiarize yourself with foods that are low and high in FODMAPs, see the tables on pages 31–33.

5. "Isn't there a medication for this?"

Despite extraordinary medical advances, a medicine or miracle cure for IBS does not yet exist. Tylenol (acetaminophen) or Advil (ibuprofen) will probably not fix the problem! However, a low-FODMAP diet and certain medicines can help to better manage some of the associated symptoms.

Here are a few tips to help a person suffering from irritable bowel syndrome:

- Learn more about IBS. (Reading this book is a good start!)
- Offer your help in everyday situations or periods of crisis.
- Encourage the person suffering from IBS to follow a low-FODMAP diet and support them in their efforts.

What can I drink?

Water is by far the best choice. You can add a few slices of lemon, other fruits or vegetables to flavor it to your taste. Be careful with teas and herbal infusions, as some contain FODMAPs. Green, white and black tea, as well as peppermint tea, are all low in FODMAPs.

During the reintroduction phase, how long does it take to know whether a food causes symptoms?

It can take anywhere from a couple of hours to 2 days for symptoms to show up, depending on the food and the time it takes to be digested.

Keeping a food journal can help you discover which foods are responsible for your symptoms.

What should I do if the FODMAP approach doesn't work for me?

This approach is effective in 75% of cases. For the other 25%, the results are modest or nonexistent. In some cases, poor results may be due to the diet not being followed properly, but it's also possible that foods other than FODMAPs are the cause of the gastrointestinal symptoms. Keeping a food journal can help you discover which foods are responsible. People suffering from IBS who haven't seen positive results from a low-FODMAP diet are advised to work on their anxiety by applying relaxation techniques.

Making the Low-FODMAP Diet Easier

Following the low-FODMAP diet means altering your recipes and paying more attention when buying ingredients and when eating out. Here are some tips to ease the application of this diet in your daily life.

How to Adapt Your Own Recipes

To follow a low-FODMAP diet, you will need to change the ingredients you cook with, but the final result can be just as flavorful. Make the most of herbs and spices as replacements for onions and garlic: they add flavor and aroma to meals, plus they enable you to reduce added salt, thereby decreasing your risk of cardiovascular disease.

Changes in Dietary Guidelines for IBS Since the Adoption of the Low-FODMAP Approach

	PREVIOUS RECOMMENDATIONS	CURRENT RECOMMENDATIONS
Fruits and vegetables	Reduce or eliminate gas-forming foods, such as broccoli, cauliflower, cabbage, beans and carrots. If necessary, eat cooked fruits and vegetables rather than raw, to ease digestion.	It's no more a matter of avoiding gas-forming foods. Now it's the high-FODMAP fruits and vegetables that must be avoided.
Chewing gum, soft drinks and sweeteners	Avoid chewing gum, soft drinks and carbonated water because they increase the amount of air swallowed and cause bloating.	On top of previous recommendations, which are still valid, avoid foods that use the following sweeteners: mannitol, sorbitol and xylitol.
Lactose	No specific guidelines, unless one is lactose-intolerant.	Minimize the intake of high-lactose foods during the elimination phase.
Fiber	For constipation, increase insoluble fiber (wheat, bran cereals, bread, whole-grain pasta, brown rice, etc.). For diarrhea, increase soluble fiber (oats, barley, rye, legumes, etc.).	Whole grains are still recommended because they are part of a healthy diet. However wheat, rye and barley should be avoided during the elimination phase, as they all contain fructans.

If you feel you just can't live without the taste of garlic, simply prepare a garlic-infused oil (see recipe, page 147) or use garlic scapes, which you can find fresh in markets during the spring or canned in delicatessens at any time of year.

Onions, leeks and shallots do need to be eliminated as ingredients, and it's also important to make sure they are not hidden in premade foods such as spice mixes, stocks and broths, sauces, marinades and so on. Even a tiny amount of onion contains a large amount of fructan, which can pass into other ingredients and cause symptoms. To give your dishes a mild onion flavor, you can use the green part of green onions and chives, added right at the end of cooking. Or, if you can find some, young onion shoots contribute a lot of flavor without a lot of fructan. You should confirm your individual level of tolerance.

How to Spot FODMAPs on Food Labels

Avoiding individual high-FODMAP foods, such as apples, honey or wheat, is rather simple. What's more complicated is figuring out whether a food or dish consisting of several ingredients is low or high in FODMAPs. For example, how do you choose a bread or breakfast cereal? In such cases, you need to know how to interpret the list of ingredients.

The ingredients lists that appear on food packaging may seem complicated, since they tend to use a lot of unfamiliar words. To make your job easier and help you make the right low-FODMAP choices for you, here is a list of ingredients that contain FODMAPs:

- agave syrup
- chicory root
- dried fruits
- fruit juice concentrate
- garlic powder (or any other garlic flavoring)
- high-fructose corn syrup
- honey
- inulin
- isomalt
- legume flours
- maltitol
- mannitol
- onion powder (or any other onion flavoring)
- polydextrose
- sorbitol
- xylitol

The fact that FODMAPs are fermentable carbohydrates (sugars) explains why most of the above ingredients are used as sweeteners! But the good news is that a low-FODMAP diet need not be devoid of all sugars and/or carbs. Here is a list of sweeteners that are usually well tolerated:

- brown rice syrup
- brown sugar
- cane sugar
- corn syrup
- dextrose
- glucose
- granulated (white) sugar
- maple syrup
- powdered (icing) sugar
- stevia
- sucrose

Also bear in mind that the earlier an ingredient appears in the list of ingredients, the greater the amount of that ingredient in the food.

How to Make the Best Choices When Eating Out

Ideally, avoid going to restaurants during the elimination phase. In time, you will be comfortable enough with the FODMAP approach to choose the right dishes when eating out: you'll simply need to bring the detachable page containing helpful lists of allowed foods and those to avoid. Many restaurants now offer gluten-free options, so explain to your server that you also need your dish to be free of garlic and onions. The table opposite offers a selection of low-FODMAP choices from various types of restaurants.

In any case, even if you make a small exception in your diet and experience symptoms, you can always get back on track.

How to Travel without Worry

You may think it's impossible to travel without any issues if you suffer from IBS, but that's not the case! Read on to discover our best tips for an enjoyable vacation.

Establish and Maintain a Routine

This may be easier said than done, but it's worth trying nonetheless. Your body is used to a particular routine, so try to stick to it as much as possible, even when travelling internationally or through different time zones. If you aren't able to maintain a perfect routine during your trip, that's okay: you are on holiday to have fun, so make the most of it!

Best Low-FODMAP Choices When Eating Out

Asian	Sashimi and sushi (as long as they don't contain high-FODMAP ingredients such as avocado or asparagus)
	Fried rice or stir-fried rice noodles with vegetables (ask for a preparation with no onions, shallots or garlic and check the sauces)
	Avoid tempura dishes, as tempura is made from wheat
Breakfast/brunch	Omelet (made with lactose-free milk or almond milk) with low-FODMAP vegetables served with cubed potatoes and gluten-free bread
Indian	Kebabs, tikka and tandoori dishes served with white rice
Italian	Gluten-free pasta with marinara sauce, carbonara sauce or garlic-free pesto
	Grilled meat, poultry or fish with polenta and steamed or grilled vegetables
	Pizza with a gluten-free crust, tomato sauce and low-FODMAP toppings of choice
Mexican	Corn chips, beef or chicken tacos, tamales, tostadas, fajitas, nachos (avoid guacamole, beans and other legumes)
Pub food	Grilled or roasted meat, poultry or fish with low-FODMAP vegetables (avoid hamburgers, as they may contain high-FODMAP ingredients)
	Main-course salads

Stick with the Elimination Phase

A vacation isn't the best time to try new foods. Even if you are ready for the reintroduction phase, it is better to delay your food tests and continue with the elimination phase during your trip. The change of scenery could distort the food test results and compromise your return to a more varied diet.

One good tip is to bring with you the dry goods you're used to eating for breakfast. Cereals or packets of oatmeal, for example, will help you start the day right. In most hotels, you'll have access to a fridge, so take a trip to the local supermarket and stock up on low-FODMAP fruits for your breakfasts and snacks. And if you're lucky enough to have access to a kitchen, why not prepare some meals yourself? In addition to saving a little money, you'll be certain of what you're eating, which will give your intestines some rest.

If you plan to eat out a lot while on vacation, see the table above for the best options at various restaurants.

Reduce Your Stress Level

Although this recommendation is useful at all times and for everyone, it is even more important for someone with IBS who is traveling. You can reduce your stress levels during your trip by planning your activities and itineraries in advance.

DID YOU KNOW?

Managing Stress with Exercise

If you haven't already done so, include physical activity in your everyday life. In addition to its many benefits to your physical health, exercise helps you better manage periods of stress (such as when you are traveling) and to detach from the stresses of day-to-day life. Add exercise to your routine and stick with it when you're on holiday.

No matter how well you plan, however, unexpected and stressful surprises tend to be par for the course when it comes to vacations. There are many ways to manage stress, and they are all equally effective, as long as they work for you. Visualization, meditation and yoga are some of the best stress-management tools.

Be Ready in Case of Emergency

Even with extraordinary planning, emergencies can happen. Once again, preparation plays a key role. Make sure you have the right tools at hand to manage the situation, including travel insurance. In addition, let the people you're traveling with know that you have a condition that can cause certain intestinal urgencies. IBS is one of the most common illnesses, so don't be surprised if you're not the only one struggling with it. You'll be able to exchange tips with those in the same boat.

How to Survive Year-End Holidays

If you suffer from IBS, any holiday event or party can easily become unpleasant. Many party foods are high in fat and contain onions and garlic, so bloating, cramps and tummy aches are never far behind. Thankfully, there are easy ways to ensure that you have a wonderful festive season without any bad memories! Here are a few tips and tricks.

Planning: The Key to Success

It is important to remember that it isn't the end of the world if your special-occasion dinner isn't 100% low-FODMAP. With FODMAPs, it's all about balance and quantity. If you know you're going to be eating away from home, plan ahead and reduce your intake of FODMAPs for the rest of the day. This will give you a wider variety of choice.

If you're invited to a potluck meal, why not bring a dish that's low in FODMAPs? That way, you're sure to have something that's safe for you to eat. If possible, ask other participants to write the ingredients of their dish on a small card. This will take them only a few moments and could save you a lot of discomfort. What's more, it will also be useful for anyone else suffering from food allergies or dietary intolerances!

Even when a party isn't a potluck, don't hesitate to ask your hosts if you can bring your own dish. They are sure to appreciate that they don't need to worry about dietary restrictions when planning the meal.

> If you know you're going to be eating away from home, plan ahead and reduce your intake of FODMAPs for the rest of the day.

Beverage Consumption

- **Avoid high-FODMAP alcohol:** Most mixed drinks and cocktails should be avoided, as they are generally high in FODMAPs. If you simply must have a piña colada or a daiquiri, check the ingredients and avoid those that contain FODMAP-rich ingredients. Rum and sweet wines should also be avoided, as they contain an excess of fructose compared to their glucose content.
- **Go for low-FODMAP drinks:** Wine (red, rosé and white), sparkling wine (Champagne, cava), beer, vodka and whiskey are all low in FODMAPs. A note on sparkling wine: any drink with bubbles should be consumed sparingly, given that the ingestion of air can produce symptoms, especially bloating.
- **Be careful!** Even low-FODMAP alcohol cannot be consumed freely. Alcohol in general is an irritant for the digestive system and can cause symptoms such as bloating and diarrhea. Our favorite tip? Alternate each alcoholic drink with a glass of something nonalcoholic and low in FODMAPs (see the examples in the sidebar). Not only will you be properly hydrated and avoid excess alcohol, you will also protect your digestive system.

DID YOU KNOW?

Low-FODMAP Non-Alcoholic Drinks
When you want to drink something other than alcohol, homemade lemonade or water with a few slices of cucumber (or any mix of low-FODMAP fruits and/or vegetables) can be a great choice.

General Tips to Cope with the Holidays

- Don't skip meals, and try to eat at regular times. It is not advisable to fast during the day simply so you can indulge and eat too much at the party.
- Stick to your usual routine as much as possible and take time to do some physical activity.
- Go for a long walk — this can work miracles when it comes to relieving stress!

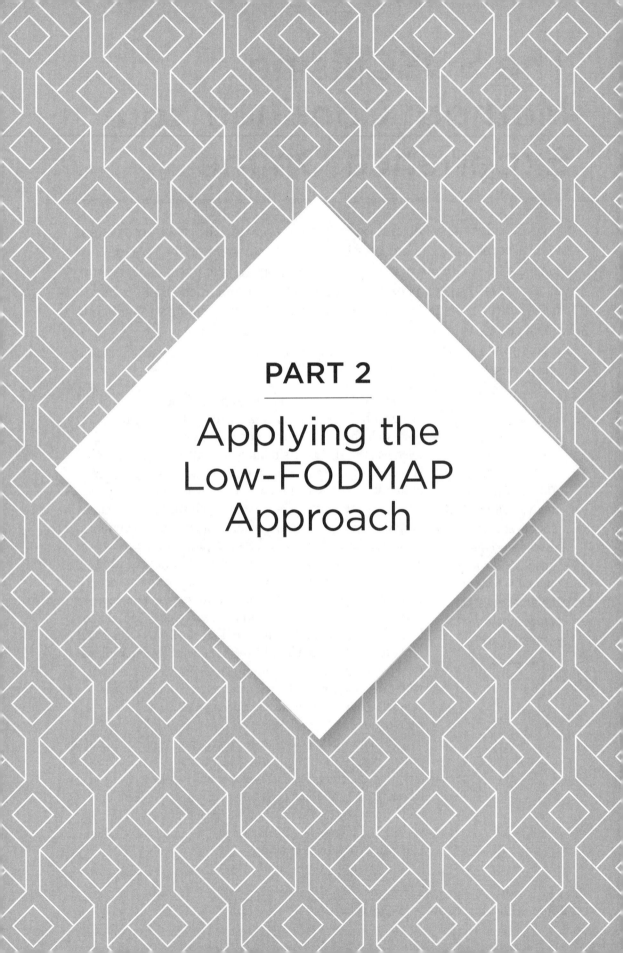

PART 2

Applying the
Low-FODMAP
Approach

The SOSCuisine Method: Continue Your Experience Online

Changing your dietary habits is never easy, even when you're very motivated, because ingrained habits can be a big obstacle to change. In the case of adopting a low-FODMAP diet, there's the additional challenge of dealing with lists of allowed foods and excluded foods. What's more, foods that seem very similar, from a botanical or flavor point of view, are sometimes very different when it comes to their FODMAP content. For example, you can eat raspberries without problems, as they do not contain FODMAPs, but you cannot consume blackberries, as they contain polyols.

The meal plans and recipes in parts 2 and 3 of this book, along with all the information, advice and tips in part 1, are there to help you adopt this diet and identify your individual tolerance threshold. To simplify your task even further as you get started, we invite you to continue your experience online at www.soscuisine.com. There, you will find complete low-FODMAP meal plans, renewed each week, with recipes and editable grocery lists, including upcoming discounts from your favorite supermarkets (this last feature is only available in Canada). These meal plans are designed from fresh, seasonal produce, and prepared for one to four people. You can personalize them by adding your own preferences or exclusions (for example "without beef or pork" or "gluten-free"). You'll also find hundreds of low-FODMAP recipes and other relevant advice to make the experience as enjoyable as possible for you and your family. The SOSCuisine method, with its specialized and personalized meal plans, offers a concrete answer to the eternal question "What should we eat tonight?"

> The SOSCuisine method, with its specialized and personalized meal plans, offers a concrete answer to the eternal question "What should we eat tonight?"

You can also take advantage of a support group made up of other people following the low-FODMAP diet, who share their own tips and tricks. In addition, should you so desire, you can benefit from individual coaching by a registered dietitian, who will be able to answer your questions and guide you through the food challenges. Consultations with the registered dietitian take place by phone or online.

Low-FODMAP Meal Plans

The meal plans on the following pages will help you put the FODMAP approach into practice. They are composed of easily available ingredients from the four food groups — fruits and vegetables, grain products, milk and substitutes, and meat and substitutes. Furthermore, these meal plans are well balanced and nutritionally adequate.

You may change the amounts depending on your personal needs, but you will need to pay attention to the total FODMAP content you consume on a daily basis. Feel free to repeat the meal plans, exchange one meal for another and make your own combinations.

Low-FODMAP Meal Plan: Week 1

	SUNDAY	MONDAY	TUESDAY
Breakfast	• 1 slice gluten-free bread + 1 tbsp (15 mL) almond butter • ¾ cup (175 mL) gluten-free cereal + 1 tsp (5 mL) ground flax seeds (flaxseed meal) + ½ cup (125 mL) enriched almond milk • 1 orange (6 oz/ 180 g)	• ⅔ cup (150 mL) lactose-free yogurt + ⅓ cup (75 mL) Homemade Granola* • 1 slice gluten-free bread + 1 tbsp (15 mL) peanut butter • 1 small banana (5 oz/ 150 g)	• Oatmeal* + 1 cup (250 mL) lactose-free milk • 1 slice gluten-free bread + 1 slice (⅓ oz/10 g) lactose-free cheese • 2 clementines (4 oz/ 120 g)
Morning snack	• ½ cup (125 mL) lactose-free yogurt + ⅓ cup (75 mL) raspberries	• Homemade Microwave Popcorn*	• ¾ cup (175 mL) grapes • 7 almonds
Lunch	• My Grandma's Cream of Tomato Soup* • Quinoa and Pecan Salad* • Berry Tofu Mousse*	• Turkey and Cheese Sandwich* • Grated Carrot Salad* • 1 kiwifruit (3 oz/ 90 g) • 1 cup (250 mL) lactose-free milk	• Watercress Soup* • Mixed Vegetable Salad with Eggs* • 1 slice gluten-free bread • Small Bowl of Strawberries and Raspberries*
Afternoon snack	• 1 cup (250 mL) green tea	• 1 square dark chocolate (1 oz/ 30 g)	• 1 rice cake • 1 oz (25 g) Cheddar cheese
Dinner	• Salmon with a Spicy Crust* • Potato and Arugula Salad* • 1 slice gluten-free bread • ¾ cup (175 mL) grapes	• Chicken Piccata* • Sautéed Carrots* • Steamed Millet*	• Romaine Lettuce with a Creamy Vinaigrette* • Provence-Style Cod Casserole* • 1 slice gluten-free bread • 1 orange (6 oz/ 180 g)

* The recipe appears in the book; the portion size is 1 serving unless otherwise indicated.

WEDNESDAY	THURSDAY	FRIDAY	SATURDAY
• Strawberry-Banana Smoothie with Tofu* • 2 slices gluten-free bread + 2 tbsp (30 mL) peanut butter	• Oatmeal* + 1 cup (250 mL) lactose-free milk • 1 slice gluten-free bread + 1 slice (⅓ oz/10 g) lactose-free cheese • 2 passion fruits (4 oz/120 g)	• 1 slice gluten-free bread + 1 tbsp (15 mL) almond butter • ¾ cup (175 mL) gluten-free cereal + 1 tsp (5 mL) ground flax seeds (flaxseed meal) + ½ cup (125 mL) enriched almond milk • ½ cup (125 mL) cubed cantaloupe	• Buckwheat Pancake with Egg* • 1 cup (250 mL) lactose-free milk • 2 clementines (4 oz/ 120 g)
• ⅓ cup (75 mL) walnuts (1 oz/ 30 g)	• 10 hazelnuts	• 1 cup (250 mL) lactose-free milk • 1 small banana (5 oz/150 g)	• ½ cup (125 mL) lactose-free yogurt + 1 kiwifruit (3 oz/90 g)
• Rice and Lentil Salad with Herbs* • Tomato and Feta Cheese Salad* • 1 kiwifruit (3 oz/ 90 g) • 1 cup (250 mL) enriched almond milk	• Vegetable Salad with Mackerel* • 1 oz (25 g) Emmental cheese • Quick Berry Sorbet*	• Pork Chops with a Mustard Sauce* • Potato Purée with Olive Oil* • Oven-Roasted Peppers*	• Baked Tofu with Ginger* • Braised Bok Choy* • Steamed Millet* • Lemon Polenta Cake*
• ½ cup (125 mL) lactose-free yogurt + ⅓ cup (75 mL) grapes	• ½ cup (125 mL) lactose-free yogurt + ⅓ cup (75 mL) blueberries	• 1 small carrot • 1 tbsp (15 mL) sunflower seeds	• 1 square dark chocolate (1 oz/ 30 g)
• Kale and Orange Salad* • Beef Stew en Papillote* • Okra with Tomatoes* • Steamed Brown Rice*	• My Grandma's Cream of Tomato Soup* • Chicken Saltimbocca* • Skillet Endive* • Steamed Brown Rice* • ¾ cup (175 mL) grapes	• Bacon, Lettuce and Tomato Penne* • Berry Tofu Mousse*	• Asian Beef and Vegetable Soup* • 2 slices gluten-free crispbread • ½ dragon fruit (7 oz/200 g)

Low-FODMAP Meal Plan: Week 2

	SUNDAY	MONDAY	TUESDAY
Breakfast	• 1 cup (250 mL) rice puffs + 10 hazelnuts + 1 tsp (5 mL) ground flax seeds (flaxseed meal) + 1 cup (250 mL) enriched almond milk • 1 slice gluten-free bread + 1 tbsp (15 mL) almond butter • 1 small banana (5 oz/150 g)	• 2 slices gluten-free bread + 2 tsp (10 mL) non-hydrogenated margarine + 2 slices smoked salmon • ½ grapefruit (5 oz/ 150 g) • 1 cup (250 mL) lactose-free milk	• ⅔ cup (175 mL) lactose-free yogurt + ⅓ cup (75 mL) Homemade Granola* • 1 slice gluten-free bread + 1 tbsp (15 mL) peanut butter • ¾ cup (175 mL) grapes
Morning snack	• 1 cup (250 mL) green tea	• Chickpea Muffin*	• 1 rice cake • 1 oz (25 g) Gruyère cheese
Lunch	• Carrot Soup with Orange and Ginger* • Shrimp and Arugula Quinoa Salad*	• Turkey and Cheese Sandwich* • Kale and Orange Salad* • 4 Brazil nuts	• Carrot Soup with Orange and Ginger* • Egg Salad Sandwich* • Tomato Salad with Oregano*
Afternoon snack	• Berry, Maple and Yogurt Parfait*	• 1 cup (250 mL) green tea	• Strawberry-Banana Smoothie with Tofu*
Dinner	• Blackened Fish Fillets* • Greek-Style Roasted Vegetables* • 2 slices gluten-free crispbread • Cucumber and Tomato Salad*	• Roasted Peppers with Tomatoes* • Thai Noodles with Beef* • Kiwi and Orange Sabayon Gratin*	• Provence-Style Chicken* • Potato Purée with Olive Oil* • 1 slice gluten-free bread

* The recipe appears in the book; the portion size is 1 serving unless otherwise indicated.

WEDNESDAY	THURSDAY	FRIDAY	SATURDAY
• 1 cup (250 mL) rice puffs + 2 tbsp (30 mL) walnuts + 1 tsp (5 mL) ground flax seeds (flaxseed meal) + 1 cup (250 mL) lactose-free milk • 1 slice gluten-free bread + 1 tbsp (15 mL) almond butter • 1 kiwifruit (3 oz/ 90 g)	• Oatmeal* + 1 cup (250 mL) lactose-free milk • 1 slice gluten-free bread + 1 slice (⅓ oz/10 g) lactose-free cheese • 2 passion fruits (120 g)	• Cantaloupe Smoothie* • Cinnamon-Scented Quinoa*	• 1 fried egg • 2 slices gluten-free bread • 3 slices canned pineapple • 1 cup (250 mL) lactose-free milk
• Allergy-Friendly Banana Bread*	• Strawberry-Banana Smoothie with Tofu*	• Two-Colored Fruit Salad*	• 1 slice gluten-free crispbread + 1 oz (25 g) Brie cheese
• Grilled Chicken Caesar Salad* • 1 slice gluten-free bread • 1 cup (250 mL) lactose-free milk	• Winter Vegetable Soup* • Mixed Vegetable Salad with Eggs*	• Poached Eggs and Smoked Ham in an Orange Sauce* • Mixed Greens with Classic Vinaigrette* • 1 slice gluten-free bread	• Prosciutto-Wrapped Pork Tenderloin* • Spinach with Raisins* • Steamed Brown Rice* • Sugared Oranges*
• ½ cup (125 mL) cubed honeydew melon	• 2 clementines (4 oz/120 g)	• ½ cup (125 mL) lactose-free yogurt + ⅓ cup (75 mL) raspberries	• ½ cup (125 mL) lactose-free yogurt + 1 kiwifruit (3 oz/90 g)
• Winter Vegetable Soup* • Tofu Burger* • ½ cup (125 mL) lactose-free yogurt + ⅓ cup (75 mL) raspberries	• Watercress and Orange Salad* • Lamb Shanks with Potatoes* • 1 slice gluten-free bread	• Blue Cheese Turkey Burger* • Boston Lettuce, Tomato and Radish Salad* • Quinoa Pudding*	• Chicken Fajitas* + Tomato and Cucumber Salsa* • Small Bowl of Strawberries and Raspberries*

Low-FODMAP Meal Plan: Week 3

	SUNDAY	MONDAY	TUESDAY
Breakfast	• Oatmeal* + 1 cup (250 mL) lactose-free milk • 1 slice gluten-free bread + 1 slice (⅓ oz/10 g) lactose-free cheese • 2 clementines (4 oz/ 120 g)	• Green Tea Smoothie* • 2 slices gluten-free bread + 2 tbsp (30 mL) peanut butter	• Cinnamon-Scented Quinoa* + 1 tsp (5 mL) ground flax seeds (flaxseed meal) • ½ grapefruit (5 oz/ 150 g) • 1 cup (125 mL) lactose-free milk
Morning snack	• ½ cup (125 mL) lactose-free yogurt + ⅓ cup (75 mL) blueberries	• ¾ cup (175 mL) grapes • 1 cup (250 mL) enriched almond milk	• 1 tbsp (15 mL) sunflower seeds • 1 cup (250 mL) enriched almond milk
Lunch	• Watercress and Orange Salad* • Flemish Beef Stew* • 1 slice gluten-free bread • Tapioca Pudding*	• Warm Quinoa and Arugula Salad* • Quick Berry Sorbet*	• Egg Salad Sandwich* • Roasted Peppers with Tomatoes* • 1 small banana (5 oz/150 g)
Afternoon snack	• 1 cup (250 mL) green tea	• Chickpea Muffin*	• 1 rice cake + 1 tbsp (15 mL) almond butter
Dinner	• Asian Shrimp Soup* • Prosciutto and Kiwi* • 2 slices of gluten-free crispbread	• Japanese-Style Chicken Skewers* • ½ cup (125 mL) blanched broccoli • Steamed Basmati Rice* • Tapioca Pudding*	• Radish and Cucumber Salad* • Filet Mignon with a Creamy Paprika Sauce* • Greek-Style Roasted Vegetables* • 1 slice gluten-free bread • Two-Colored Fruit Salad*

* The recipe appears in the book; the portion size is 1 serving unless otherwise indicated.

WEDNESDAY	THURSDAY	FRIDAY	SATURDAY
• 1 slice gluten-free bread + 1 tbsp (15 mL) peanut butter • ¾ cup (175 mL) gluten-free cereal + 1 tsp (5 mL) ground flax seeds (flaxseed meal) + ½ cup (125 mL) enriched almond milk • ½ cup (125 mL) cubed honeydew melon	• Cantaloupe Smoothie* • 2 slices gluten-free bread + 2 slices (each ⅓ oz/10 g) lactose-free cheese	• 1 slice gluten-free bread + 1 tbsp (15 mL) almond butter • ¾ cup (175 mL) gluten-free cereal + 1 tsp (5 mL) ground flax seeds (flaxseed meal) + ½ cup (125 mL) enriched almond milk • ½ grapefruit (5 oz/ 150 g)	• Cinnamon-Scented Quinoa* + 1 tsp (5 mL) ground flax seeds (flaxseed meal) • ½ cup (125 mL) cubed papaya • 1 cup (125 mL) lactose-free milk
• 1 rice cake + 1 oz (25 g) mozzarella cheese	• 1 small carrot • 2 radishes	• ½ cup (125 mL) lactose-free yogurt + 4 Brazil nuts	• 1 kiwifruit (3 oz/ 90 g)
• Parsnip and Potato Soup* • Chicken Salad with a Coriander-Mustard Dressing* • 1 slice gluten-free bread • 3 slices canned pineapple	• Ham and Cheese Sandwich* • Mixed Greens and Strawberry Salad* • Tofu Mousse with Peanut Butter*	• Baked Salmon with Herbs* • Spinach with Raisins* • Steamed Basmati Rice*	• Curried Trout* • Mint Zucchini* • Steamed Millet* • Rice Pudding*
• ¾ cup (175 mL) grapes	• 1 square dark chocolate (1 oz/ 30 g)	• ¾ cup (175 mL) blueberries	• Allergy-Friendly Banana Bread*
• Tomato and Green Bean Salad* • Singapore Noodles* • 1 orange (6 oz/ 180 g)	• Grilled Chicken in Coconut Milk with Spices* • Braised Bok Choy* • Mashed Potatoes* • ½ dragon fruit (7 oz/ 200 g)	• Vegetable Fritters* • Spaghetti with Citrus Pesto*	• Parsnip and Potato Soup* • Ratatouille with Tofu* • Steamed Brown Rice*

Vegan Low-FODMAP Meal Plan

	SUNDAY	MONDAY	TUESDAY
Breakfast	• Green Tea Smoothie* • 2 slices gluten-free bread + 2 tbsp (30 mL) peanut butter	• Cantaloupe Smoothie* • Cinnamon-Scented Quinoa*	• 1 cup (250 mL) rice puffs + 10 hazelnuts + 1 tsp (5 mL) ground flax seeds (flaxseed meal) + 1 cup (250 mL) enriched almond milk • 1 slice gluten-free bread + 1 tbsp (15 mL) almond butter • 1 small banana (5 oz/150 g)
Morning snack	• Chickpea Muffin*	• 1 rice cake + 1 tbsp (15 mL) almond butter	• Chickpea Muffin*
Lunch	• Rice and Lentil Soup* • Wheat-Free Tabbouleh* • 1 slice gluten-free bread	• Rice and Lentil Salad with Herbs* • Tomato Salad with Oregano* • 1 slice gluten-free bread • Ginger-Flavored Rhubarb Sorbet*	• Rice and Lentil Soup* • Wheat-Free Tabbouleh* • 2 slices gluten-free crispbread
Afternoon snack	• 1 small banana (5 oz/150 g) • 1 tbsp (15 mL) almonds	• 2 tbsp (30 mL) walnuts • 1 cup (250 mL) enriched almond milk	• ⅓ cup (75 mL) walnuts (1 oz/30 g)
Dinner	• Baked Tofu with Ginger* • Braised Bok Choy* • 1 slice gluten-free bread • 2 tbsp (30 mL) sunflower seeds • Ginger-Flavored Rhubarb Sorbet*	• Baked Tofu with Ginger* • Braised Bok Choy* • 1 slice gluten-free bread • Small Bowl of Strawberries and Raspberries* • ⅓ cup (75 mL) walnuts (1 oz/30 g)	• My Grandma's Cream of Tomato Soup* • Tofu Burger* • Grilled Vegetables* • Berry Tofu Mousse*

* The recipe appears in the book; the portion size is 1 serving unless otherwise indicated.

WEDNESDAY	THURSDAY	FRIDAY	SATURDAY
• 1 cup (250 mL) rice puffs + 10 hazelnuts + 1 tsp (5 mL) ground flax seeds (flaxseed meal) + 1 cup (250 mL) enriched almond milk • 1 slice gluten-free bread + 1 tbsp (15 mL) almond butter • 1 small banana (5 oz/150 g)	• Cantaloupe Smoothie* • Cinnamon-Scented Quinoa*	• 1 slice gluten-free bread + 1 tbsp (15 mL) peanut butter • ¾ cup (175 mL) gluten-free cereal + 1 tsp (5 mL) ground flax seeds (flaxseed meal) + ½ cup (125 mL) enriched almond milk • ½ cup (125 mL) cubed honeydew melon	• 1 cup (250 mL) rice puffs + 10 hazelnuts + 1 tsp (5 mL) ground flax seeds (flaxseed meal) + 1 cup (250 mL) enriched almond milk • 1 slice gluten-free bread + 1 tbsp (15 mL) almond butter • 1 small banana (5 oz/150 g)
• Homemade Microwave Popcorn*	• 1 cup (250 mL) green tea	• 2 tbsp (30 mL) walnuts • 1 cup (250 mL) enriched almond milk	• Homemade Microwave Popcorn*
• Rice and Lentil Salad with Herbs* • Tomato Salad with Oregano* • 1 slice gluten-free bread • Berry Tofu Mousse*	• Indian-Style Tofu Sauté* • Steamed Millet* • Grilled Vegetables*	• Asian Vegetable Soup* • Mixed Greens with Classic Vinaigrette*	• Asian Vegetable Soup* • Mixed Greens with Classic Vinaigrette*
• Chickpea Muffin*	• Tofu Mousse with Peanut Butter*	• Small Bowl of Strawberries and Raspberries*	• 1 rice cake + 1 tbsp (15 mL) peanut butter
• Indian-Style Tofu Sauté* • Steamed Millet* • Fattoush*	• Spaghetti with Citrus and Anchovy Pesto, vegan variation* • Small Bowl of Strawberries and Raspberries*	• Tofu Burger* • Fattoush*	• My Grandma's Cream of Tomato Soup* • Sautéed Tempeh with Mixed Greens* • 1 slice gluten-free bread • Ginger-Flavored Rhubarb Sorbet*

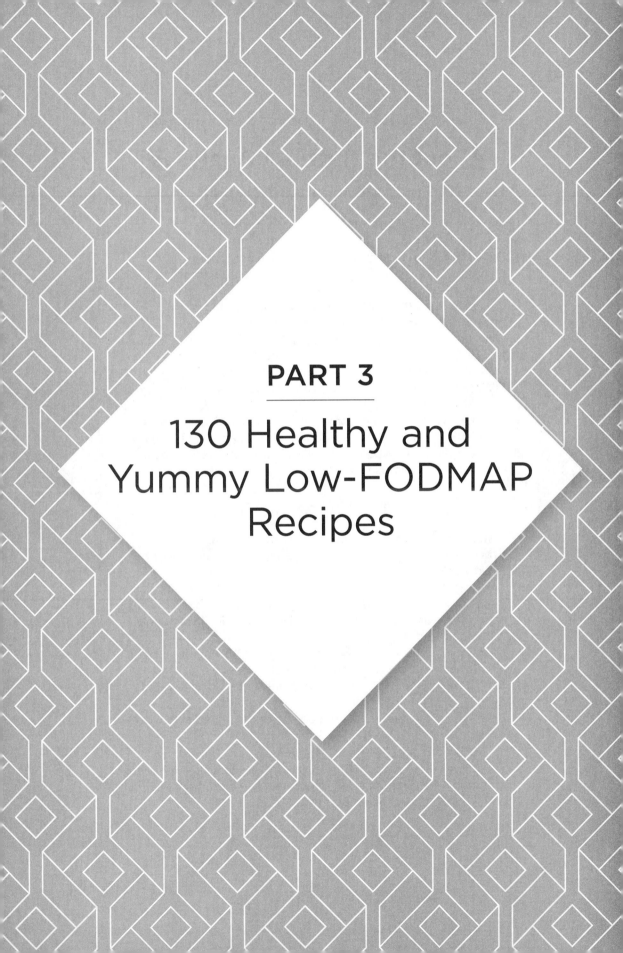

PART 3

130 Healthy and Yummy Low-FODMAP Recipes

About the Nutrient Analyses

The nutrient analyses were derived from the SOSCuisine.com proprietary Nutrition Analysis Software, which uses information from the following databases:

1. Banca Dati di Composizione degli Alimenti per Studi Epidemiologici in Italia (2015). Retrieved June 2016 from www.bda-ieo.it.
2. Canadian Nutrient File (2012). Retrieved June 2016 from https://food-nutrition.canada.ca/cnf-fce/index-eng.jsp.
3. Fineli Food Composition Database (2016). Retrieved June 2016 from https://fineli.fi/fineli/en/elintarvikkeet.
4. Monash University (2015). The Monash University Low FODMAP Diet (version 1.4) [Mobile App]. Downloaded from http://itunes.apple.com.
5. Standard Tables of Food Composition in Japan (2015). Retrieved June 2016 from http://database.food.sugiyama-u.ac.jp/index_asia.php.
6. USDA Food Composition Databases (2015). Retrieved June 2016 from https://ndb.nal.usda.gov/ndb.

Recipes were evaluated as follows:

- All calculations were based on ingredient weights.
- Where alternatives are given, the first ingredient and amount listed were used.
- Optional ingredients and ingredients that are not quantified were not included in the calculations, with the exception of salt, which was calculated as a pinch where a specific amount is not indicated.
- Nutrient values are rounded to the nearest whole number for calories, protein, carbohydrates, fiber and sodium. Nutrient values are rounded to one decimal point for fat and saturated fat.
- Calculations took into account cooking of the ingredients where possible.

It is important to note that the cooking method used, ingredient substitutions and differences among brand-name products may alter the nutrient content per serving.

Breakfasts and Snacks

Homemade Granola

**MAKES
36 SERVINGS
(ABOUT
$\frac{1}{3}$ CUP/75 ML
PER SERVING)**

· MAKE AHEAD ·

· FREEZABLE ·

Preparation time:

10 minutes

Cooking time:

35 minutes

*This granola is much
healthier than store-
bought types, which
contain preservatives,
refined sugars and too
much fat. It's also tastier
and cheaper.*

TIP
The granola will keep
for several weeks in the
refrigerator or up to
3 months in the freezer.

NUTRIENTS PER SERVING

Calories	140
Protein	4 g
Fat	6.0 g
Saturated fat	2.0 g
Carbohydrates	18 g
Fiber	3 g
Sodium	2 mg

- **Preheat oven to 375°F (190°C)**
- **Large rimmed baking sheet, oiled**

8 cups	large-flake (old-fashioned) rolled oats	2 L
1 cup	unsweetened flaked coconut	250 mL
1¾ cups	hazelnuts, coarsely chopped	425 mL
¼ cup	canola oil	60 mL
⅓ cup	pure maple syrup	75 mL

1. Combine the oats, coconut and hazelnuts in a large bowl. Pour the oil and syrup over the dry ingredients, then toss well. Spread the mixture onto the prepared baking sheet.

2. Bake in the middle of the preheated oven for 30 to 40 minutes or until golden brown and crispy. Stir every 10 minutes to brown evenly and avoid burning the mixture.

3. Let the granola cool down; it will become crispier and dry as it cools. Make sure to break up any large clumps of granola while the mixture is still warm. Once it has completely cooled, transfer it to an airtight container or plastic bag.

Oatmeal

**MAKES
1 SERVING**

Preparation time:

5 minutes

Cooking time:

10 minutes

You can add plenty of low-FODMAP toppings to this basic oatmeal recipe. Peanut butter, a few slices of banana and a couple of dark chocolate chips make for a fun breakfast!

⅓ cup	large-flake (old-fashioned) rolled oats	75 mL
Pinch	salt	Pinch
⅔ cup	water	150 mL

1. Combine the oats, salt and water in a saucepan. Bring it all to a boil, stirring, then remove from heat, cover and let sit for about 5 minutes, so that there will be some "chew" to it. Serve.

NUTRIENTS PER SERVING

Calories	120
Protein	4 g
Fat	2.0 g
Saturated fat	0.4 g
Carbohydrates	21 g
Fiber	3 g
Sodium	4 mg

Poached Eggs and Smoked Ham in an Orange Sauce

Preparation time:

15 minutes

Cooking time:

40 minutes

Usually served for a brunch, but equally appreciated in other occasions.

TIP
Keep the serving plates in the oven at the lowest setting so they are warm when you serve.

NUTRIENTS PER SERVING	
Calories	400
Protein	23 g
Fat	22.0 g
Saturated fat	7.0 g
Carbohydrates	25 g
Fiber	3 g
Sodium	980 mg

Potato Pancakes

2	potatoes (14 oz/400 g total)	2
2	large eggs	2
¼ cup	lactose-free cream (any fat level)	60 mL
¼ cup	chopped fresh dill	60 mL
	Salt and freshly ground black pepper	
1 tbsp	canola oil	15 mL

Poached Eggs

1 tbsp	white wine vinegar	15 mL
4	large eggs	4

Orange Sauce

1	medium orange	1
2 tbsp	non-hydrogenated margarine	30 mL
¼ cup	white wine	60 mL
¼ cup	lactose-free cream	60 mL
2 tbsp	Cointreau or Grand Marnier liqueur (optional)	30 mL
4	slices smoked ham (about 9 oz/260 g)	4
1 tsp	finely chopped fresh chives	5 mL

1. *Potato Pancakes:* Boil the potatoes in their skins in a saucepan of water until they are soft, about 15 to 20 minutes depending on their size. Drain the potatoes and peel them while they are still warm. Place the potatoes in a bowl and mash them until they become puréed.

2. Beat 2 eggs, then add them to the potatoes. Pour in the cream. Stir in the chopped dill, season with salt and pepper and mix well. Chill the mixture for a few minutes, until it becomes firm, then divide it into 4 pancakes.

The potato pancakes
can be prepared a few
days in advance. Store
the cooked pancakes in
an airtight container
in the refrigerator, then
reheat in the oven or a
skillet before assembly.

3. Meanwhile, preheat oven to 170°F (77°C).

4. Heat the oil in a heavy skillet over medium-high heat. When the pan is hot, add the potato pancakes and cook them for 3 to 4 minutes per side, turning them once, until they are golden-brown. Transfer the pancakes to a plate and keep them warm in the oven.

5. *Poached Eggs:* Fill a medium saucepan with about 3 inches (7.5 cm) water. Bring it to a boil, add vinegar, then reduce the heat to keep the liquid barely simmering.

6. Crack each egg into a separate small cup. Gently lower the lip of each egg cup $\frac{1}{2}$ inch (1 cm) below the water surface and let the egg flow out. Immediately cover the pan and turn off the heat. Cook the eggs for 3 minutes for medium-firm yolks. Lift each perfectly poached egg from the water with a slotted spoon and place it on a towel to let any water clinging to the egg drain off.

7. *Orange Sauce:* Grate the zest of the orange, then peel it and cut the fruit into bite-size pieces. Melt the margarine in a pan over medium-high heat. Add the zest and orange pieces and sweat for 2 minutes. Pour in the wine and reduce until it has evaporated. Pour in the cream and Cointreau (if using). Cook for a few minutes to reduce to the desired consistency for a sauce. Set aside.

8. *Assembly:* Put 1 potato pancake on each warmed plate. Arrange a ham slice on top of each pancake and place the poached egg on top. Pour the sauce over the egg, sprinkle with chives and serve.

Buckwheat Pancakes with Eggs

Preparation time:

10 minutes

Standing time:

2 hours

Cooking time:

10 minutes

This gluten-free recipe is ideal for breakfast, or serve it as a light lunch with a salad.

½ cup	buckwheat flour	125 mL
¼ tsp	salt	1 mL
¼ tsp	baking soda	1 mL
¾ cup	water	175 mL
2 tsp	canola oil	10 mL
1 tsp	non-hydrogenated margarine	5 mL
2	large eggs	2

1. Combine the flour, salt, baking soda and water in a bowl. Mix well, using a whisk, until the texture is smooth. Let stand in the refrigerator about 1 to 2 hours to obtain a lighter texture.

2. Preheat oven to 170°F (77°C).

3. Oil a nonstick frying pan and put it over medium heat. Pour about ¼ to ⅓ cup (60 to 75 mL) of the batter onto the center of the pan. Spread it rapidly, either by whirling the pan or using a spatula. After about 2 minutes, when the pancake turns golden-brown, flip it and cook for 1 more minute. Keep the cooked pancake warm in the oven. Repeat with the remaining batter to make 1 more pancake.

4. Meanwhile, heat the margarine in another pan over medium-low heat and cook the eggs sunny-side up or as desired. Place one egg on top of each pancake then serve.

NUTRIENTS PER SERVING	
Calories	230
Protein	11 g
Fat	11.0 g
Saturated fat	2.5 g
Carbohydrates	25 g
Fiber	2 g
Sodium	420 mg

Cinnamon-Scented Quinoa

VEGAN

**MAKES
1 SERVING**

· MAKE AHEAD ·

· FREEZABLE ·

Preparation time:

5 minutes

Standing time:

5 minutes

Cooking time:

15 minutes

An excellent way to fill up with energy in the morning.

TIP

Cooked quinoa can be refrigerated in an airtight container for up to 3 days or frozen for up to 3 months; thaw before reheating, if necessary.

NUTRIENTS PER SERVING	
Calories	220
Protein	5 g
Fat	4.5 g
Saturated fat	0.3 g
Carbohydrates	42 g
Fiber	3 g
Sodium	60 mg

¼ cup	quinoa	60 mL
½ cup	water	125 mL
1	cinnamon stick	1
Pinch	salt	Pinch
2 tsp	walnuts	10 mL
½ tbsp	raisins	7 mL
1 tbsp	pure maple syrup	15 mL
¼ cup	unsweetened fortified almond milk	60 mL

1. Place the quinoa in a fine-mesh strainer and hold it under cold running water until the water runs clear, then drain well.

2. Combine the quinoa, water, cinnamon stick and salt in a saucepan. Bring to a boil, then reduce to a simmer. Cover and cook until the grains are translucent and the germ has spiraled out from each grain, about 15 minutes.

3. Remove pan from heat and let stand, covered, for 5 minutes. Remove the cinnamon stick, fluff with a fork, then pour into a bowl. (The cinnamon stick can be rinsed, dried and stored for reuse in another recipe.) Top with walnuts, raisins, maple syrup and almond milk, then serve.

Cantaloupe Smoothie

 VEGAN

**MAKES
1 SERVING**

Preparation time:

10 minutes

*Smoothies are a quick
and easy way to increase
your fruit consumption.
Make sure to choose a
fortified soy milk made
from soy protein only
(low-FODMAP) and
not from whole soybeans
(high-FODMAP).*

TIP

For a thicker smoothie,
increase the amount
of tofu and reduce
the milk.

• **Blender or food processor**

½ cup	diced ripe cantaloupe	125 mL
1 cup	unsweetened fortified soy milk, made with soy protein	250 mL
¼ tsp	vanilla extract	1 mL
¼ cup	soft tofu	60 mL

1. Place the cantaloupe in the blender or food processor. Add the milk and vanilla. Process on the highest speed until a well-blended purée forms, about 15 seconds, stopping to scrape down the sides of the container once or twice. Incorporate the tofu, then serve.

NUTRIENTS PER SERVING

Calories	180
Protein	15 g
Fat	4.5 g
Saturated fat	2.0 g
Carbohydrates	21 g
Fiber	1 g
Sodium	150 mg

Green Tea Smoothie

VEGAN

MAKES 1 SERVING

Preparation time:

5 minutes

TIP

To increase the protein content, soy milk may be substituted for the almond milk. Make sure to choose a fortified beverage made from soy protein only (low-FODMAP) and not from whole soybeans (high-FODMAP).

- **Blender or food processor**

1	ripe banana	1
½ tsp	matcha (fine powder green tea), or more to taste	2 mL
2 tsp	pure maple syrup	10 mL
¼ cup	soft tofu	60 mL
1 cup	unsweetened fortified almond milk	250 mL

1. Crush the banana on a little dish and mix in the matcha. Transfer the mixture to the blender or food processor. Add the maple syrup, tofu and almond milk. Process on the highest speed until a well-blended purée forms, about 1 or 2 minutes. Serve.

NUTRIENTS PER SERVING

Calories	200
Protein	6 g
Fat	6.0 g
Saturated fat	0.4 g
Carbohydrates	35 g
Fiber	3 g
Sodium	200 mg

Strawberry-Banana Smoothie with Tofu

**MAKES
1 SERVING**

Preparation time:

10 minutes

TIPS

For a denser smoothie, increase the amount of tofu and reduce the milk.

If fresh strawberries are off season, don't hesitate to use frozen ones.

- **Blender or food processor**

½	ripe banana, broken into chunks	½
½ cup	strawberries	125 mL
1 cup	lactose-free milk	250 mL
¼ cup	soft tofu	60 mL

1. Place the banana chunks and strawberries in the blender or food processor. Add the milk. Process on the highest speed until a well-blended purée forms, about 15 seconds, stopping to scrape down the sides of the container once or twice. Incorporate the tofu, then serve.

Vegan Variation

Unsweetened fortified almond milk or soy milk (made from soy protein) may be substituted for the lactose-free milk.

NUTRIENTS PER SERVING	
Calories	210
Protein	15 g
Fat	5.0 g
Saturated fat	2.0 g
Carbohydrates	28 g
Fiber	3 g
Sodium	140 mg

Berry, Maple and Yogurt Parfait

Preparation time:

5 minutes

TIP

For an added protein boost, use lactose-free Greek yogurt instead of lactose-free yogurt.

7 tbsp	plain lactose-free yogurt	105 mL
1/3 cup	strawberries or blueberries	75 mL
1 tbsp	pure maple syrup	15 mL
1	serving Homemade Granola (page 70)	1

1. Layer yogurt, strawberries, maple syrup and granola in a cup and serve.

NUTRIENTS PER SERVING

Calories	280
Protein	8 g
Fat	9.0 g
Saturated fat	4.0 g
Carbohydrates	42 g
Fiber	4 g
Sodium	60 mg

Tofu Mousse with Peanut Butter

**MAKES
1 SERVING**

• MAKE AHEAD •

Preparation time:

5 minutes

TIP

Be careful to choose soft tofu and not silken tofu. Silken tofu is high in FODMAPs! See page 36 for more details on the FODMAP-content of soy foods.

• **Blender**

¾ cup	soft tofu (about 6½ oz/190 g)	175 mL
2 tbsp	natural peanut butter	30 mL
1 tbsp	pure maple syrup (approx.)	15 mL
⅛ tsp	vanilla extract	0.5 mL

1. Put the tofu in the blender. Add the peanut butter, maple syrup and vanilla. Process on the highest speed until a creamy consistency is obtained, about 2 minutes.

2. Pour the mixture into a bowl and serve.

NUTRIENTS PER SERVING	
Calories	300
Protein	19 g
Fat	16.0 g
Saturated fat	3.0 g
Carbohydrates	29 g
Fiber	4 g
Sodium	190 mg

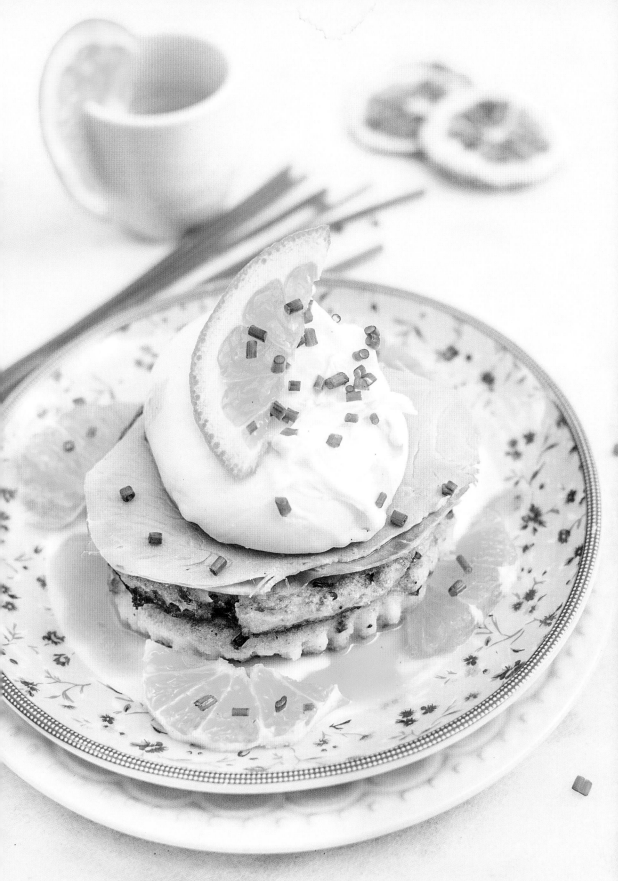

Poached Eggs and Smoked Ham in an Orange Sauce (page 72)

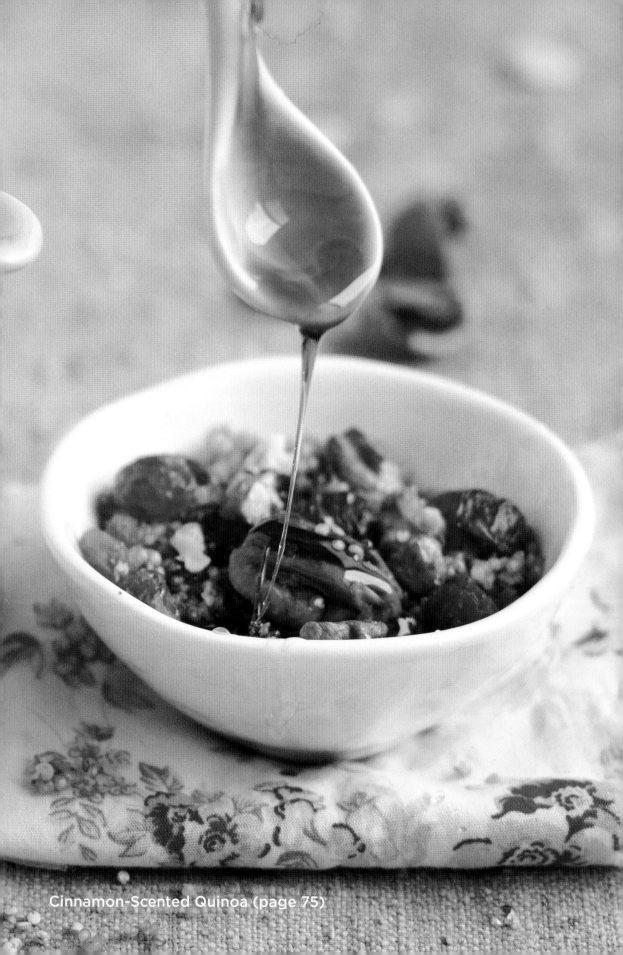

Cinnamon-Scented Quinoa (page 75)

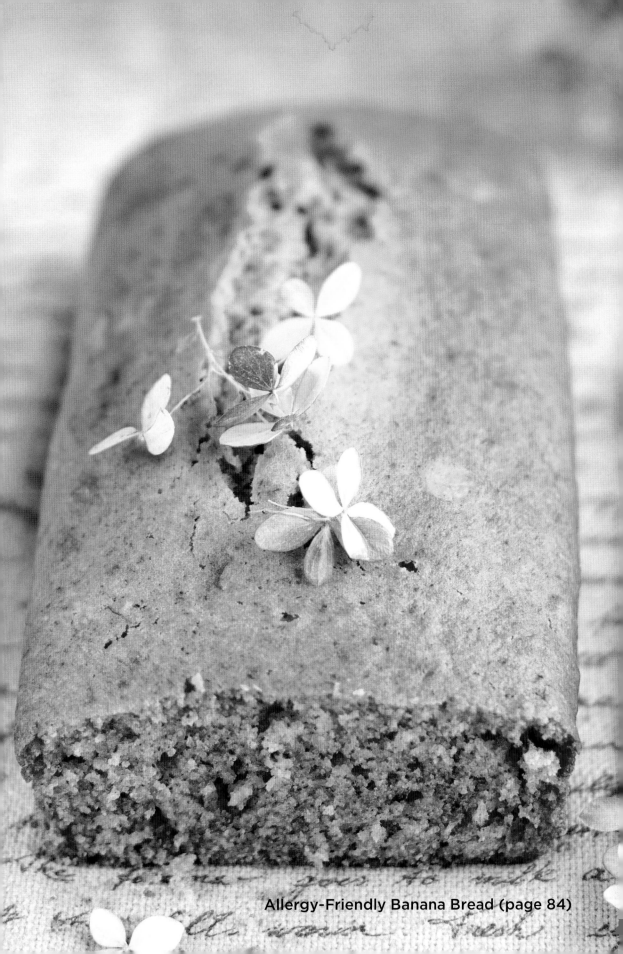

Allergy-Friendly Banana Bread (page 84)

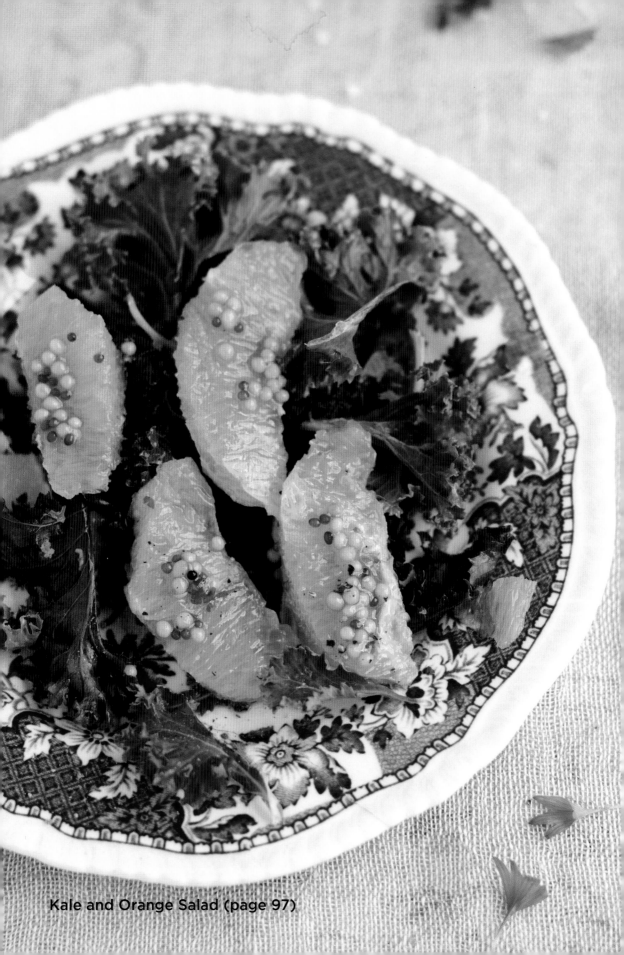

Kale and Orange Salad (page 97)

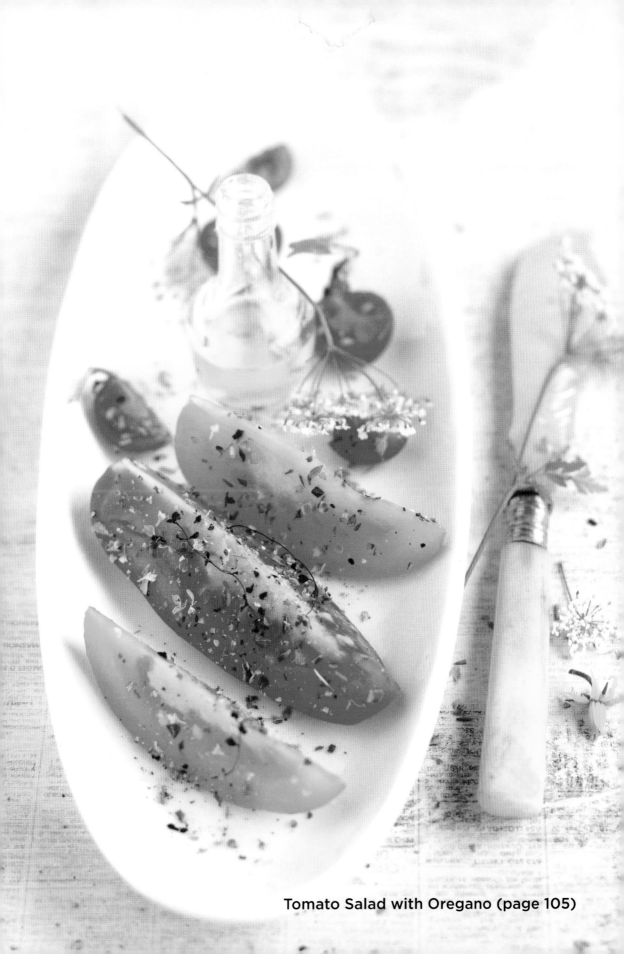

Tomato Salad with Oregano (page 105)

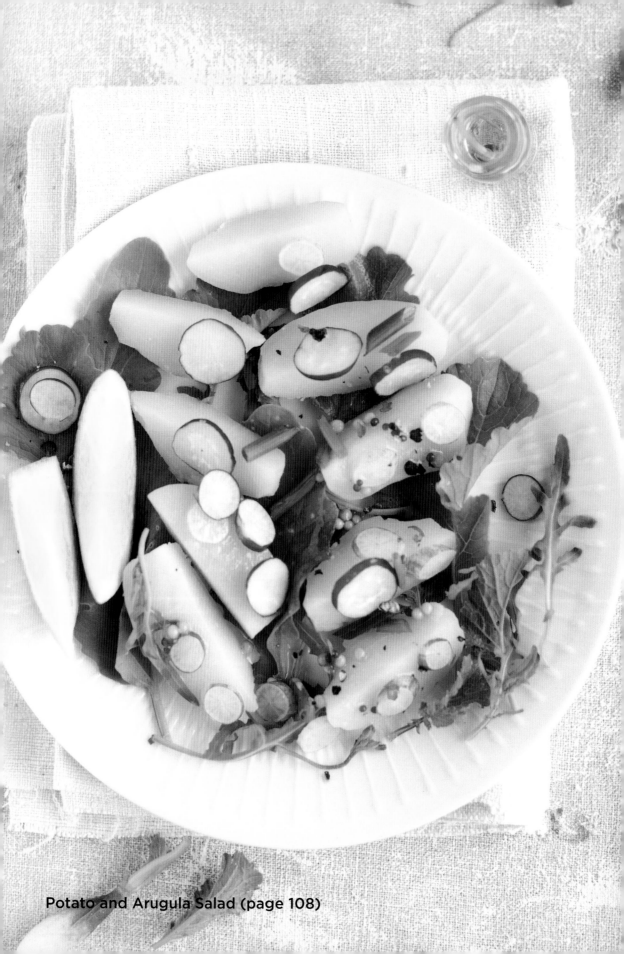

Potato and Arugula Salad (page 108)

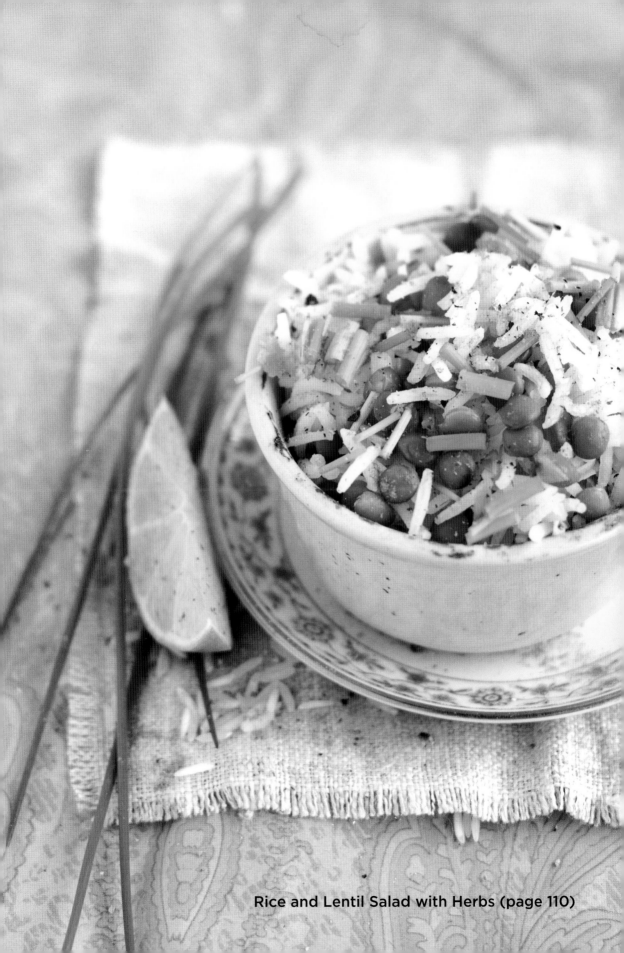

Rice and Lentil Salad with Herbs (page 110)

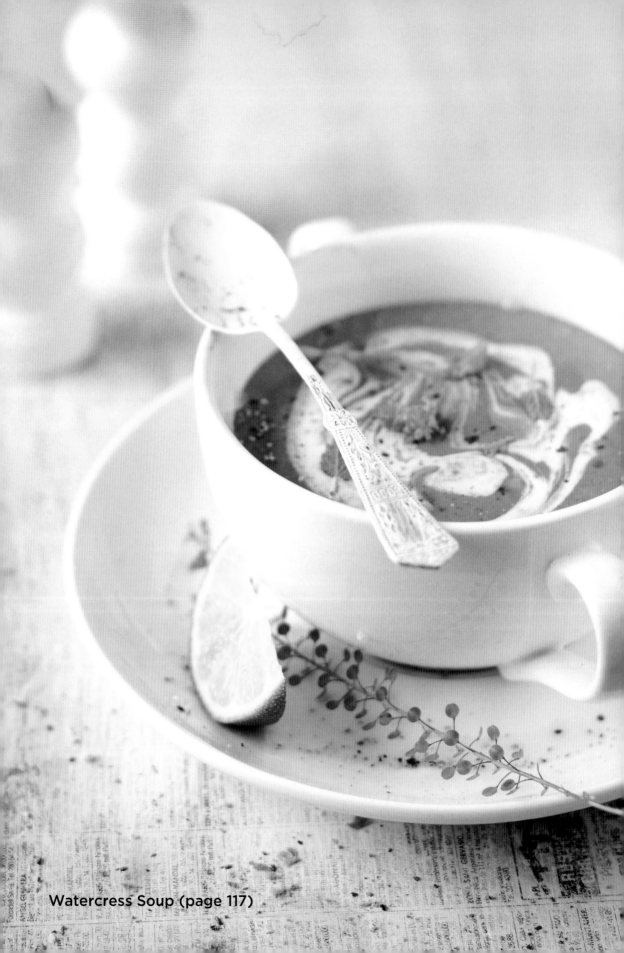

Watercress Soup (page 117)

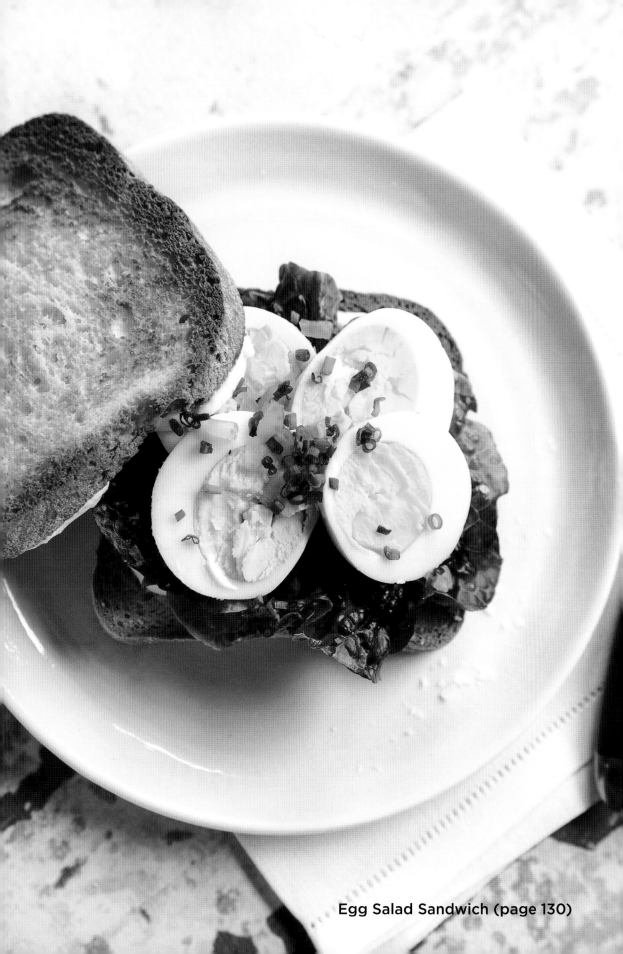

Egg Salad Sandwich (page 130)

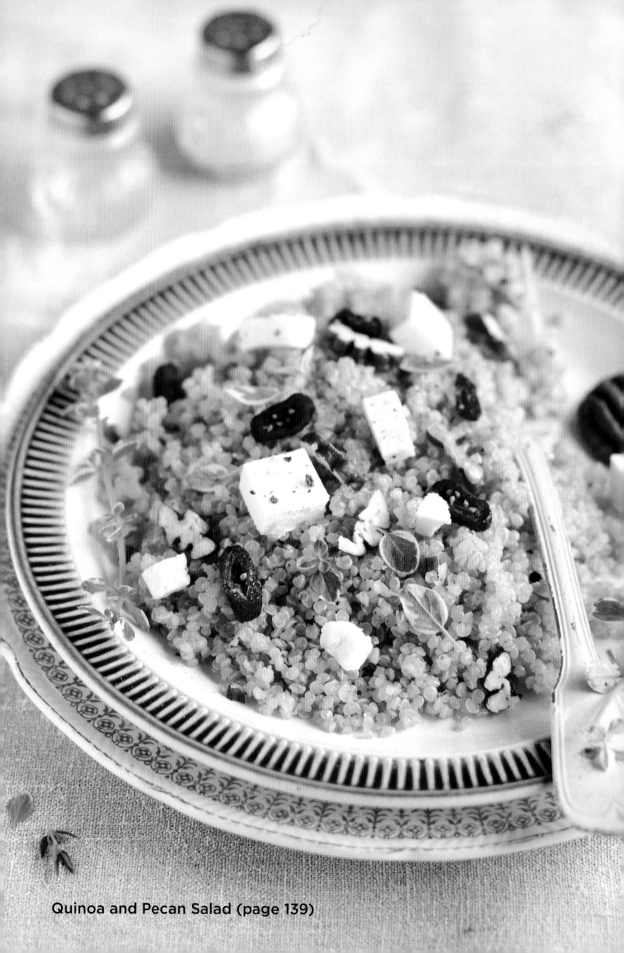

Quinoa and Pecan Salad (page 139)

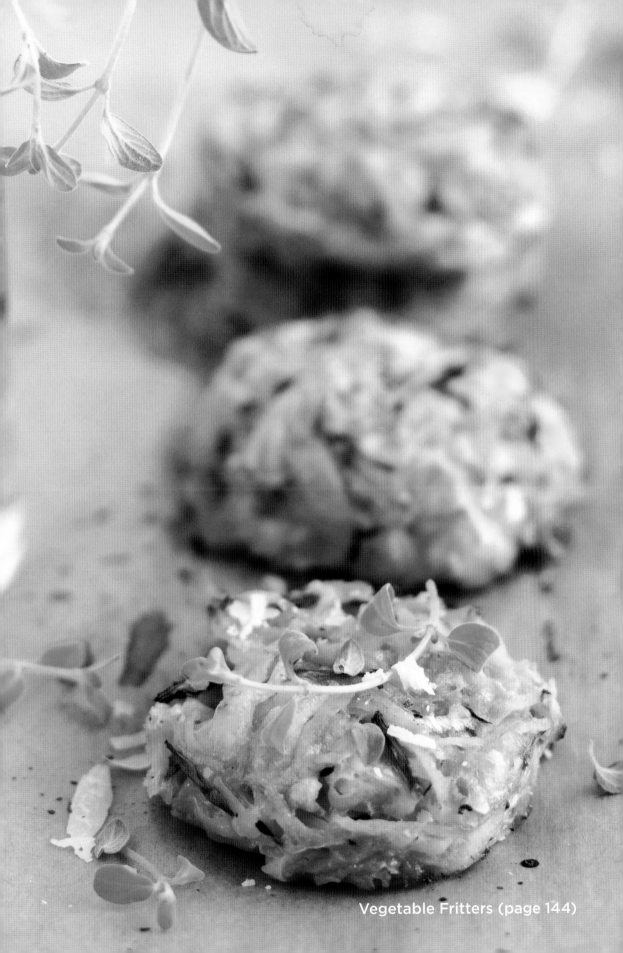

Vegetable Fritters (page 144)

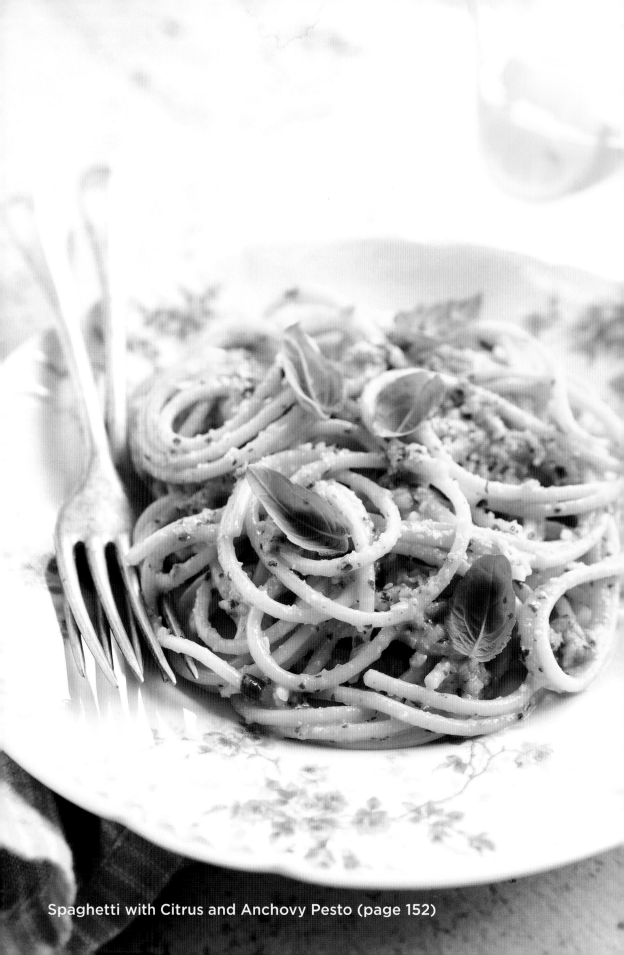

Spaghetti with Citrus and Anchovy Pesto (page 152)

Homemade Microwave Popcorn

**MAKES
2 SERVINGS**

· MAKE AHEAD ·

Preparation time:

2 minutes

Cooking time:

3 minutes

Homemade popcorn is easy and far cheaper than throwing a bag of processed popcorn into the microwave. Best of all, you can control the type and amount of seasoning.

TIP

Cooled popcorn can be stored in an airtight container at room temperature for up to 2 days.

NUTRIENTS PER SERVING

Calories	110
Protein	3 g
Fat	2.5 g
Saturated fat	0.4 g
Carbohydrates	20 g
Fiber	4 g
Sodium	2 mg

- **Microwave-safe bowl**
- **Vented microwave food cover**

1 tsp	extra virgin olive oil	5 mL
Pinch	salt	Pinch
¼ cup	popcorn kernels	60 mL
2 tsp	herbes de Provence	10 mL

1. Put the olive oil and salt in microwave-safe bowl. Use a bowl that is large enough to contain all the popped kernels (¼ cup/60 mL kernels yields about 6 cups/ 1.5 L of popped popcorn). If you use a glass bowl, make sure it is tempered glass and can handle the high heat. Add the popcorn kernels and stir so that the kernels get completely covered with the oil and salt mixture.

2. Cover the bowl with the vented lid. (Alternatively, you can cover the top of the bowl with parchment paper, secure it with a rubber band and poke vent holes in the top with a knife.) Microwave on High for 3 to 4 minutes or until popping slows to 1 to 2 seconds between pops. The time will vary depending on your microwave and bowl, so you may need to do some trial-and-error testing with the first few batches to figure out how long it takes the popcorn to cook.

3. Carefully remove the popcorn from the microwave oven (the bowl is hot!), sprinkle with the herbs and serve.

Cranberry Granola Bars

MAKES 12 SERVINGS

• **MAKE AHEAD** •

• **FREEZABLE** •

Preparation time:

10 minutes

Baking time:

25 minutes

Standing time:

30 minutes

These high-protein granola bars make for the perfect snack before or after exercise. They also make a good on-the-go breakfast.

• Preheat oven to 375°F (190°C)
• 8-inch (20 cm) square metal baking pan, lined with parchment paper

1½ cups	puffed rice cereal	375 mL
1¼ cups	quinoa flakes	300 mL
1¼ cups	large-flake (old-fashioned) rolled oats	300 mL
½ cup	unsweetened shredded coconut	125 mL
⅓ cup	almonds, finely chopped	75 mL
⅔ cup	dried cranberries, finely chopped	150 mL
¼ cup	flax seeds, ground	60 mL
3	large eggs	3
2 tbsp	canola oil	30 mL
6 tbsp	pure maple syrup	90 mL
¼ cup	natural almond butter	60 mL

1. In a large bowl, mix the puffed rice, quinoa flakes, oats, coconut, almonds, cranberries and flax seeds.

2. In a separate bowl, combine the eggs, oil, maple syrup and almond butter. Mix well with a whisk until smooth.

3. Add the wet mixture to the dry one, then mix well to ensure all ingredients are coated.

NUTRIENTS PER SERVING

Calories	250
Protein	7 g
Fat	12.0 g
Saturated fat	1.5 g
Carbohydrates	31 g
Fiber	4 g
Sodium	20 mg

It is also possible to bake the mixture in a muffin pan. To do so, adjust the baking time to 12 to 15 minutes.

The granola bars can be kept in an airtight container at room temperature for up to 1 week, or for a few months in the freezer.

4. Press mixture into prepared baking pan so it is compact. Bake in the middle of the preheated oven for about 25 to 30 minutes. Take the pan out of the oven, then let cool for at least 30 minutes. Cut into 12 bars, then serve.

Vegan Variation

Replace the eggs with 3 tbsp (45 mL) ground flax seeds mixed with 1 cup (250 mL) water. Let stand for 5 minutes before adding to the recipe, to allow it to gel.

Allergy-Friendly Banana Bread

VEGAN

**MAKES
16 SERVINGS**

· MAKE AHEAD ·

· FREEZABLE ·

Preparation time:

15 minutes

Baking time:

45 minutes

Standing time:

1 hour

This gluten-, dairy- and egg-free recipe is a great way to use up ripened bananas. Just put them in the freezer without peeling them and they will be there when you need them.

NUTRIENTS PER SERVING

Calories	170
Protein	2 g
Fat	6.0 g
Saturated fat	0.5 g
Carbohydrates	28 g
Fiber	2 g
Sodium	115 mg

- Preheat oven to 350°F (180°C)
- Grinder or mini chopper
- 9- by 5-inch (23 by 12.5 cm) baking dish, sprayed with nonstick vegetable oil spray

2 tbsp	flax seeds	30 mL
⅔ cup	water	150 mL
⅔ cup	hazelnuts, divided	150 mL
1¾ cups	brown rice flour (10 oz/300 g)	425 mL
½ cup	arrowroot starch	125 mL
2 tsp	baking soda	10 mL
¼ tsp	salt	1 mL
½ tsp	ground cinnamon	2 mL
¼ cup	canola oil	60 mL
⅓ cup	pure maple syrup	75 mL
3	very ripe bananas, mashed (1 lb/460 g)	3
1 tbsp	freshly squeezed lemon juice	15 mL

1. Grind the flax seeds and place them in a bowl or cup. Stir in water and let stand for 5 minutes to gel. Set aside.

2. Finely grind half of the hazelnuts and chop the remaining half. Put the ground hazelnuts in a large bowl. Add the rice flour, arrowroot, baking soda, salt and cinnamon, then mix well.

3. In a separate bowl, combine the oil and maple syrup. Add the flax seed mixture, bananas, and lemon juice, mixing well. Add this wet mixture to the dry mixture and stir until just moistened, without overmixing. Fold in the chopped hazelnuts with a spatula.

TIPS

If arrowroot starch is not available, replace it with about $\frac{1}{3}$ cup (75 mL) cornstarch.

Store cooled bread, tightly wrapped at room temperature, for up to 2 days or freeze for up to 3 months.

4. Transfer the batter to the prepared baking dish. Bake in the middle of the preheated oven for about 45 minutes or until the bread is done. Check for doneness with a toothpick or knife to see if the bread is cooked through.

5. Pull the baking dish out of the oven and let stand at least 30 minutes before removing the bread from the dish. After removing the bread, let it cool on a wire rack for at least an additional 30 minutes before serving.

Chickpea Muffins

**MAKES
12 SERVINGS**

· MAKE AHEAD ·

· FREEZABLE ·

Preparation time:

15 minutes

Baking time:

20 minutes

*The addition of
cardamom gives a nice
flavor to these healthy
and delicious muffins.*

NUTRIENTS PER SERVING	
Calories	180
Protein	5 g
Fat	7.0 g
Saturated fat	1.0 g
Carbohydrates	24 g
Fiber	2 g
Sodium	140 mg

- Preheat oven to 325°F (160°C)
- Blender or food processor
- Electric mixer
- 12-cup muffin pan, lined with paper liners

1¾ cups	rinsed drained canned chickpeas	425 mL
2 tbsp	freshly squeezed lemon juice	30 mL
	Grated zest of ½ orange	
3 tbsp	freshly squeezed orange juice	45 mL
¼ cup	canola oil	60 mL
½ cup	granulated sugar, divided	125 mL
2	large eggs	2
3	cardamom pods	3
½ cup	quinoa flour, sifted	125 mL
⅓ cup	almond meal (ground almonds)	75 mL
2 tsp	baking powder	10 mL
⅛ tsp	salt	0.5 mL

1. Purée the chickpeas in the blender or food processor. Add the lemon juice, orange zest, orange juice, oil and all but 1 tbsp (15 mL) of the sugar. Separate the egg whites from the yolks: add the yolks to the blender, add the whites to a bowl. Purée the chickpea mixture until smooth.

2. Remove the cardamom seeds from the pods, then crush the seeds using a bottle or a meat tenderizer. Mix a pinch of cardamom with the reserved sugar, then set aside. Put the remaining cardamom in a bowl with the flour, almond meal, baking powder, and salt, then mix well. Incorporate the chickpea mixture into the flour mixture.

3. Using the mixer, beat the egg whites to stiff peaks, then fold them into the mixture, blending gently with a spatula.

Cooled muffins can be stored in an airtight container at room temperature for up to 2 days or individually wrapped, then placed in an airtight container, and frozen for up to 2 months.

4. Using an ice cream scoop, spoon the batter into the prepared muffin cups. Sprinkle each muffin with the sugar-cardamom mixture.

5. Bake in the middle of the preheated oven for about 18 to 20 minutes, until a toothpick inserted into the center of a muffin comes out clean. Take the pan out of the oven and put each of the paper-lined muffins on a rack to cool. Serve.

Vegan Variation

Replace the eggs with 2 tbsp (30 mL) ground flax seeds mixed with $2/3$ cup (150 mL) water. Let stand for 5 minutes before adding to the recipe, to allow it to gel.

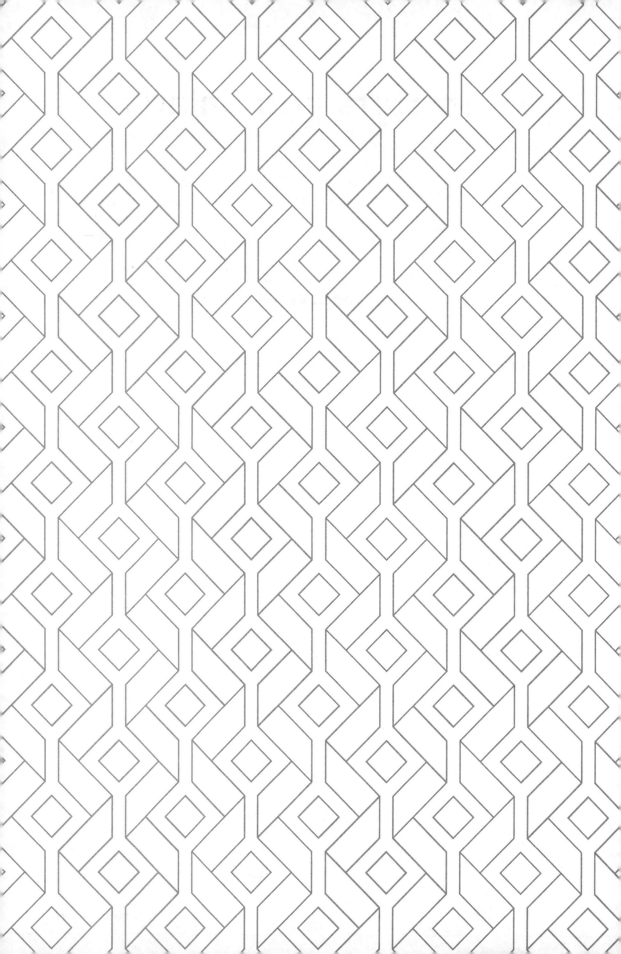

Starters and Salads

Prosciutto and Kiwi

Preparation time:

5 minutes

This is a winter version of the Italian classic Prosciutto and Cantaloupe. Kiwis are a champion of antioxidants and vitamins C and K, and are also high in dietary fiber.

TIP

When buying the prosciutto, have it sliced very thin (paper-thin), as its taste will then be at its best. Also, you will get more slices for the same price!

| 4 | kiwifruit | 4 |
| 18 | very thin slices prosciutto (about 7 oz/200 g) | 18 |

1. Peel the kiwi and slice it. Arrange the prosciutto and the kiwi slices on a platter or on individual plates. Serve.

NUTRIENTS PER SERVING	
Calories	120
Protein	15 g
Fat	2.5 g
Saturated fat	0.5 g
Carbohydrates	12 g
Fiber	2 g
Sodium	630 mg

Tomato and Cucumber Salsa

MAKES 4 SERVINGS

Preparation time:

10 minutes

Standing time:

15 minutes

A nice and speedy salsa that can be made more or less spicy according to your taste.

1	medium cucumber, diced	1
	Salt	
4	plum (Roma) tomatoes	4
3 tbsp	olive oil	45 mL
2 tsp	wine vinegar	10 mL
	Freshly ground black pepper	
$1/2$ tsp	hot pepper sauce, such as Tabasco (or to taste)	2 mL
1 tbsp	chopped fresh cilantro (optional)	15 mL

1. Sprinkle the cucumbers with salt and let drain about 15 minutes. Rinse and pat dry.

2. Meanwhile, dice the tomatoes, discarding the seeds. Put them in a salad bowl. Add cucumbers to the bowl.

3. In a small bowl, beat the oil and vinegar, using a fork, until well combined. Season with salt and pepper. Add the Tabasco sauce. For a more exotic flavor, add a few chopped cilantro leaves, but be careful with the amount, since it may be overpowering.

4. Pour dressing over the salad. Let stand for a few minutes before serving.

NUTRIENTS PER SERVING

Calories	110
Protein	1 g
Fat	11.0 g
Saturated fat	1.5 g
Carbohydrates	4 g
Fiber	1 g
Sodium	10 mg

Roasted Peppers with Tomatoes

VEGAN OPTION

MAKES
4 SERVINGS

• MAKE AHEAD •

Preparation time:

15 minutes

Cooking time:

10 minutes

TIPS

Instead of grilling or broiling, the peppers can be roasted whole on a rimmed baking sheet in a 425°F (220°C) oven for 30 minutes.

To make the salad ahead, prepare through step 3, cover and refrigerate for up to 8 hours.

NUTRIENTS PER SERVING

Calories	270
Protein	3 g
Fat	24.0 g
Saturated fat	3.5 g
Carbohydrates	13 g
Fiber	3 g
Sodium	340 mg

• **Preheat barbecue grill to high or preheat broiler**

2	yellow or red bell peppers	2
4	medium tomatoes, sliced	4
12	black olives	12
6	oil-packed sun-dried tomatoes, drained and chopped	6
3	anchovy fillets, drained and chopped	3
1 tbsp	drained capers	15 mL
1 tbsp	pine nuts	15 mL
1/3 cup	extra virgin olive oil	75 mL
1 tbsp	balsamic vinegar	15 mL
1 tbsp	freshly squeezed lemon juice	15 mL
1 tbsp	Parsley Base (see recipe, opposite)	15 mL
2 tbsp	chopped fresh chives	30 mL
	Salt and freshly ground black pepper	

1. Cut the peppers into quarters lengthwise and remove the seeds and stalks. Cook, skin side down, over the hot grill or on a rimmed baking sheet under the broiler for about 5 minutes, until the skin chars. Turn over and cook for 2 to 3 minutes. Transfer to a bowl and let cool for a few minutes.

2. Peel the peppers and cut them into strips lengthwise, then arrange them on a serving dish. Arrange tomatoes on the serving dish with the peppers. Add the olives, sun-dried tomatoes, anchovies, capers and pine nuts on top of the peppers and tomatoes.

3. In a small bowl, combine the olive oil, vinegar, lemon juice and Parsley Base. Add chives to the dressing. Season with salt and pepper. Whisk well, then pour the dressing over the salad and serve.

Vegan Variation

Omit the anchovies and add more capers.

Preparation time:

30 minutes

Rather than chop parsley each time a recipe calls for it, you can prepare some in advance. Make sure to use Italian parsley (also known as flat-leaf parsley) for this recipe. It is preferred to curly parsley because it is tastier and richer in essential oils. Parsley is as appealing for its vitamins and minerals as for its antioxidant potential.

TIPS

Important: To reduce the risk of food poisoning, never let the parsley base stand at room temperature.

Parsley Base can be stored in the refrigerator up to 1 month, or for 3 months in the freezer. Remember to top up with oil every time you use it, to prevent oxidation and mold formation.

Parsley Base

VEGAN

1	bunch fresh Italian (flat-leaf) parsley (3½ oz/100 g)	1
⅔ cup	olive oil	150 mL

1. Only the parsley leaves are used, as the stems are too hard. Wash and spin-dry the leaves. Finely chop them. Put them into a glass jar, cover with a layer of oil to prevent air oxidation, then put the lid on. Put the jar in the refrigerator.

Mixed Greens with Classic Vinaigrette

VEGAN

**MAKES
4 SERVINGS**

Preparation time:

5 minutes

The traditional mix includes a variety of fresh baby salad greens in a wide range of leaf shapes, colors, textures and flavors. Depending on the season, the mix might contain anywhere from a dozen to three dozen different lettuces, mostly chervil, arugula, spinach, mustard, dandelion and endive.

8 cups	mixed greens (torn, if necessary)	2 L
3 tbsp	Classic Vinaigrette (see recipe, opposite)	45 mL
	Salt and freshly ground black pepper	

1. Wash the mixed greens and blot dry. Put them in a salad bowl.
2. Pour in the Classic Vinaigrette. Add salt and pepper, toss well and serve.

NUTRIENTS PER SERVING

Calories	90
Protein	1 g
Fat	9.0 g
Saturated fat	1.0 g
Carbohydrates	2 g
Fiber	1 g
Sodium	25 mg

Preparation time:

5 minutes

Salads are often dressed at the last minute simply by adding oil, vinegar and salt, one after another, without emulsifying first. The result: one leaf is too salty, another is soaked in oil and the next is drenched with vinegar. Emulsifying the dressing before pouring it on the salad is a must, in my opinion. Besides, when you are preparing it in advance, you save time!

TIP

The vinaigrette can be kept in the refrigerator for 1 to 2 months.

Classic Vinaigrette VEGAN

³⁄₄ cup	extra virgin olive oil	175 mL
3¹⁄₂ tbsp	wine vinegar	52 mL
1 tbsp	Dijon mustard	15 mL

1. Mix the oil, vinegar and mustard in a bowl or bottle. Cover tightly and shake well for 1 minute.

Romaine Lettuce with a Creamy Vinaigrette

MAKES 4 SERVINGS

Preparation time:

10 minutes

Standing time:

1 hour

TIP

Other types of lettuce can be used in place of the romaine. Should you have any leftover lettuce, try adding it to a soup (best with Boston lettuce or curly leaf) or grill it (best with endive or romaine).

¼ cup	plain lactose-free yogurt	60 mL
1½ tsp	freshly squeezed lemon juice	7 mL
¼ tsp	Dijon mustard	1 mL
1½ tsp	chopped fresh chives	7 mL
	Salt and freshly ground black pepper	
1	head romaine lettuce (about 14 oz/400 g)	1

1. In a small bowl, mix together the yogurt, lemon juice and mustard until smooth. Add the chopped chives. Season with salt and pepper to taste. Cover and refrigerate for at least 1 hour to allow the flavors to blend.

2. Meanwhile, wash the romaine lettuce and spin-dry. Reserve the outer leaves for another use. Tear the pale green inner leaves into bite-size pieces. Put them into a salad bowl and pour in the vinaigrette. Toss and serve immediately.

NUTRIENTS PER SERVING

Calories	25
Protein	2 g
Fat	1.0 g
Saturated fat	0.3 g
Carbohydrates	4 g
Fiber	2 g
Sodium	20 mg

Kale and Orange Salad

VEGAN

2½ cups	trimmed kale leaves	625 mL
2	oranges	2
2 tbsp	extra virgin olive oil	30 mL
1 tbsp	balsamic vinegar	15 mL
1 tsp	whole-grain mustard	5 mL
	Salt and freshly ground black pepper	

MAKES 4 SERVINGS

Preparation time:

15 minutes

Cooking time:

5 minutes

1. Fill a large pot with lightly salted water, then bring to a boil. Add the kale and cook until just tender, about 3 minutes. Drain the kale and let cool slightly. Squeeze out any excess liquid then cut into large pieces and put into a salad bowl.

2. Using a sharp knife, remove the peel and pith from the oranges, then cut out the segments. Add the segments to the salad bowl.

3. In a small bowl, add the oil, vinegar and mustard. Season with salt and pepper to taste. Beat well, using a fork, until the vinaigrette is emulsified. Pour it over the salad and toss. Serve.

NUTRIENTS PER SERVING	
Calories	110
Protein	2 g
Fat	7.0 g
Saturated fat	1.0 g
Carbohydrates	11 g
Fiber	2 g
Sodium	30 mg

Mixed Greens and Strawberry Salad

Preparation time:

10 minutes

Not only do the strawberries add a touch of sweetness to this salad, they also bring in loads of antioxidants!

8 cups	mixed greens (torn, if necessary)	2 L
1 cup	strawberries, thinly sliced	250 mL
1	bocconcini (fresh mozzarella), thinly sliced (2 oz/55 g)	1
¼ cup	Classic Vinaigrette (page 95)	60 mL
1 tsp	balsamic vinegar	5 mL
	Salt and freshly ground black pepper	

1. Wash the mixed greens and blot or spin-dry. Put them in a salad bowl. Add the strawberries and bocconcini.

2. Pour in the Classic Vinaigrette and the balsamic vinegar. Add salt and pepper to taste, toss well and serve.

NUTRIENTS PER SERVING

Calories	160
Protein	4 g
Fat	15.0 g
Saturated fat	3.5 g
Carbohydrates	5 g
Fiber	2 g
Sodium	45 mg

Watercress and Orange Salad

VEGAN

MAKES 4 SERVINGS

Preparation time:

10 minutes

- Salad spinner

2	medium oranges	2
¼ cup	extra virgin olive oil	60 mL
2 tbsp	white vinegar	30 mL
2 tsp	Dijon mustard	10 mL
	Salt and freshly ground black pepper	
2	bunches watercress (about 8 oz/ 240 g)	2
½ tsp	pink peppercorns (optional)	2 mL

1. Wash, rinse and dry the orange, then remove the zest with a grater and put it in a small bowl. Pour in the oil, vinegar and mustard, then whisk well until the vinaigrette is emulsified. Add salt and pepper and set aside.

2. Rinse and spin-dry the watercress, then arrange the leaves on serving plates. Using a small knife, cut off the peel and white pith from the oranges, then cut between the membranes to separate the segments and place them on the plates. Drizzle the vinaigrette over the salad, garnish with the pink peppercorns (if using) and serve.

NUTRIENTS PER SERVING

Calories	170
Protein	2 g
Fat	15.0 g
Saturated fat	2.0 g
Carbohydrates	9 g
Fiber	2 g
Sodium	60 mg

Boston Lettuce, Tomato and Radish Salad

VEGAN

Preparation time:

10 minutes

TIP

Most types of lettuce are low in FODMAPs; you can swap out the Boston lettuce for your favorite one.

3	medium tomatoes	3
1	head Boston lettuce	1
4	radishes	4
¼ cup	Classic Vinaigrette (page 95)	60 mL
	Salt and freshly ground black pepper	

1. Cut the tomatoes into segments and place them in a salad bowl. Add the lettuce leaves. Finely slice the radish and add it to the bowl.

2. Pour in the Classic Vinaigrette. Add salt and pepper to taste. Toss and serve immediately.

NUTRIENTS PER SERVING

Calories	130
Protein	1 g
Fat	12.0 g
Saturated fat	1.5 g
Carbohydrates	5 g
Fiber	2 g
Sodium	25 mg

Grated Carrot Salad

**MAKES
4 SERVINGS**

Preparation time:

5 minutes

Carrots are a real nutritional champion, as they are packed with vitamins and minerals, including vitamin A. Their dark orange color signals the presence of carotenoids, a family of antioxidants that help in the prevention of cardiovascular diseases, certain types of cancers and certain degenerative illnesses associated with aging.

4	carrots (about 14 oz/400 g)	4
3 tbsp	Classic Vinaigrette (page 95)	45 mL
4 tsp	freshly squeezed lemon juice	20 mL
	Salt and freshly ground black pepper	

1. Peel the carrots, then shred them using a large-holed grater. Put them in a bowl.
2. Pour the Classic Vinaigrette over the carrots, add the lemon juice and season with salt and pepper. Toss to combine. Serve.

NUTRIENTS PER SERVING	
Calories	100
Protein	1 g
Fat	9.0 g
Saturated fat	1.0 g
Carbohydrates	9 g
Fiber	2 g
Sodium	70 mg

Cucumber and Tomato Salad

VEGAN

MAKES 4 SERVINGS		
2	medium cucumbers	2
	Salt	
4	medium tomatoes, sliced	2
¼ cup	Classic Vinaigrette (page 95)	60 mL
	Freshly ground black pepper	
2 tbsp	finely chopped chives	30 mL

**MAKES
4 SERVINGS**

Preparation time:

10 minutes

TIP

If you don't have any chives on hand, use green onions for a similar taste. Be sure to only use the green part, as the white part is high in FODMAPs.

1. Peel the cucumbers, slice them into rounds and sprinkle them with salt. Let them drain for a few minutes. Rinse and pat dry.

2. Arrange tomatoes on individual plates. Add the cucumbers. Pour the Classic Vinaigrette over the salad. Add salt and pepper to taste. Garnish with chopped chives and serve.

NUTRIENTS PER SERVING

Calories	140
Protein	2 g
Fat	12.0 g
Saturated fat	1.5 g
Carbohydrates	8 g
Fiber	2 g
Sodium	20 mg

Tomato and Green Bean Salad

VEGAN

	MAKES 4 SERVINGS

Preparation time:

10 minutes

Cooking time:

10 minutes

Green beans that can be eaten whole (pod and seed) are consumed as vegetables. As a matter of fact, they are a young, unripe variety belonging to a family of legumes. Not to worry, though: they are low in FODMAPs.

3 cups	green beans (10 oz/300 g)	750 mL
2	medium tomatoes	2
¼ cup	Classic Vinaigrette (page 95)	60 mL
	Salt and freshly ground black pepper	

1. Blanch the green beans for 7 to 8 minutes, until al dente. Drain and shake out the water. Set aside and let cool for a few minutes.

2. Slice the tomatoes and arrange them on individual plates. Place the beans next to the tomatoes. Sprinkle with the Classic Vinaigrette. Add salt and pepper. Serve.

NUTRIENTS PER SERVING	
Calories	140
Protein	2 g
Fat	12.0 g
Saturated fat	1.5 g
Carbohydrates	8 g
Fiber	3 g
Sodium	15 mg

Radish and Cucumber Salad

**MAKES
4 SERVINGS**

Preparation time:

10 minutes

Standing time:

15 minutes

A crunchy and refreshing salad, at its best when made with local produce.

TIP

A mandoline will make slicing easier.

2	medium cucumbers	2
	Salt	
⅓ cup	fresh dill sprigs (tough stems removed)	75 mL
12	radishes	12
2 tbsp	Classic Vinaigrette (page 95)	30 mL
	Freshly ground black pepper	

1. Cut the cucumbers into sticks and put them in a colander. Sprinkle with salt, then let drain for about 15 minutes. Rinse the cucumber sticks, drain and pat dry. Set aside.

2. Finely chop the dill and put it in a salad bowl. Cut the radishes into thin slices and add them to the bowl.

3. Add the cucumber, a little salt and pepper. Pour the Classic Vinaigrette over the salad and toss. Serve.

NUTRIENTS PER SERVING

Calories	70
Protein	1 g
Fat	6.0 g
Saturated fat	1.0 g
Carbohydrates	5 g
Fiber	1 g
Sodium	25 mg

Tomato Salad with Oregano

**MAKES
4 SERVINGS**

Preparation time:

5 minutes

*This very simple recipe
is at its best when locally
grown tomatoes are
abundant. Not only
will the tomatoes be
tastier, they will also
be richer in lycopene.
This antioxidant is
also responsible for the
tomato's red color.*

4	medium tomatoes	4
2 tbsp	extra virgin olive oil	30 mL
	Salt and freshly ground pepper	
1¾ tsp	dried oregano	8 mL

1. Cut the tomatoes lengthwise into quarters or slice them crosswise. Put them in a bowl, pour in the olive oil and season with salt and pepper. Sprinkle with oregano and toss well. Serve.

NUTRIENTS PER SERVING

Calories	80
Protein	1 g
Fat	7.0 g
Saturated fat	1.0 g
Carbohydrates	4 g
Fiber	1 g
Sodium	5 mg

Tomato and Feta Cheese Salad

Preparation time:

10 minutes

The combination of sun-ripened tomatoes and feta cheese makes a tasty salad that goes well with any grilling party.

4	medium tomatoes	4
3½ oz	feta cheese	100 g
2 tbsp	extra virgin olive oil	30 mL
12	black olives	12
1 tbsp	dried oregano	15 mL
	Freshly ground black pepper	

1. Cut the tomatoes crosswise into slices approximately ¼ inch (0.5 cm) thick and arrange them in a shallow dish.

2. Crumble the feta cheese over the tomatoes. Drizzle with oil. Add the olives and sprinkle with oregano. Season with freshly ground pepper (it is not necessary to add any salt, since the feta cheese is already rather salty). Serve at room temperature.

NUTRIENTS PER SERVING

Calories	170
Protein	5 g
Fat	14.0 g
Saturated fat	5.0 g
Carbohydrates	7 g
Fiber	2 g
Sodium	420 mg

Fattoush

Preparation time:

15 minutes

Standing time:

15 minutes

Fattoush is a rustic salad from the Middle East made with lettuce, tomatoes, cucumbers, parsley, mint and crumbled pieces of grilled pita bread. In this version, a tortilla replaces the pita.

TIP

If you cannot find sumac at your grocery store or specialty spice shop, you may substitute additional lemon juice to taste.

NUTRIENTS PER SERVING	
Calories	200
Protein	4 g
Fat	15.0 g
Saturated fat	2.0 g
Carbohydrates	16 g
Fiber	5 g
Sodium	20 mg

2	medium cucumbers	2
	Salt	
1	head romaine lettuce (about 1 lb/500 g)	1
2	medium tomatoes, coarsely diced	2
¼ cup	chopped fresh Italian (flat-leaf) parsley	60 mL
½ cup	chopped fresh mint	125 mL
¼ cup	extra virgin olive oil	60 mL
4 tsp	freshly squeezed lemon juice	20 mL
1 tbsp	ground sumac (optional)	15 mL
1	dried chile pepper, minced	1
1	6-inch (15 cm) corn tortilla	1
	Freshly ground black pepper	

1. Cut the cucumbers in half lengthwise and use a spoon to scrape out the seeds. Slice them coarsely and sprinkle them with salt to let excess and possibly bitter liquids drain off. Rinse and pat dry.

2. Wash the romaine lettuce, spin-dry, then tear the leaves into bite-size pieces. Place all the vegetables in a salad bowl or serving plate.

3. Add the oil, lemon juice, chili pepper and sumac (if using) to a small bowl. Add salt and pepper. Whisk with a fork until the vinaigrette is well combined. Adjust the seasoning. Pour over the vegetables and toss well. Let stand for 15 minutes.

4. When ready to serve, toast the tortilla in a toaster or under the broiler, break into pieces then add them to the salad. Serve.

Potato and Arugula Salad

VEGAN

Preparation time:

15 minutes

Cooking time:

15 minutes

TIP

The salad can be prepared through step 2, covered and refrigerated for up to 2 days. Let warm to room temperature before proceeding with step 3.

3	potatoes (about 1¼ lbs/600 g)	3
¼ cup	extra virgin olive oil	60 mL
1 tbsp	freshly squeezed lemon juice	15 mL
1 tbsp	Dijon mustard	15 mL
	Salt and freshly ground black pepper	
1	bunch arugula (about 5 oz/150 g)	1
1 tbsp	chopped fresh chives	15 mL
4	radishes, thinly sliced	4

1. Peel the potatoes, then cut them in half lengthwise and boil them in a pot of salted water until tender, about 15 minutes. Drain and cut each piece in half to obtain quarters. Set them aside in a bowl.

2. In a small bowl, whisk together the oil, lemon juice, mustard, salt and pepper, using a fork or whisk until the vinaigrette is emulsified. Pour the vinaigrette over the warm potatoes and toss well.

3. Wash the arugula well, then drain and place the leaves on a serving plate or in a bowl. Arrange the seasoned potatoes over the arugula, sprinkle with chopped chives and sliced radishes. Serve warm.

NUTRIENTS PER SERVING	
Calories	250
Protein	3 g
Fat	15.0 g
Saturated fat	2.0 g
Carbohydrates	26 g
Fiber	2 g
Sodium	65 mg

Wheat-Free Tabbouleh

VEGAN

Preparation time:

10 minutes

Cooking time:

15 minutes

Standing time:

10 minutes

Quinoa is the seed of a leafy plant that's related to spinach. It can substitute for rice and most other grains in side dishes, salads, soups and even puddings. It has a higher protein content than other grains and is gluten- and FODMAP-free.

6 tbsp	quinoa	90 mL
1⅓ cups	water	325 mL
	Salt	
2	bunches Italian (flat-leaf) parsley (7 oz/200 g)	2
¼ cup	fresh mint leaves	60 mL
¼ cup	finely chopped fresh chives	60 mL
¼ cup	extra virgin olive oil	60 mL
1 tbsp	freshly squeezed lemon juice	15 mL
	Freshly ground black pepper	
1	medium tomato	1

1. Place the quinoa in a fine-mesh strainer and hold it under cold running water until the water runs clear, then drain well.

2. Combine the quinoa, water and a pinch of salt in a saucepan. Bring to a boil, then reduce to a simmer. Cover and cook until the grains are translucent and the germ has spiraled out from each grain, about 15 minutes.

3. Meanwhile, wash, spin-dry and finely chop the parsley and mint leaves, discarding the larger stems. Transfer to a salad bowl along with the finely chopped chives. Toss.

4. In a small bowl, whisk together the oil and lemon juice until it is well combined. Adjust the seasoning with salt and pepper. Pour into the salad bowl, add the quinoa, then toss well. Let the salad stand for 10 minutes.

5. Dice the tomatoes, discarding the seeds, and add them to the salad; toss and serve.

NUTRIENTS PER SERVING

Calories	200
Protein	3 g
Fat	16.0 g
Saturated fat	2.0 g
Carbohydrates	13 g
Fiber	3 g
Sodium	30 mg

Rice and Lentil Salad with Herbs

MAKES 4 SERVINGS

· MAKE AHEAD ·

· FREEZABLE ·

Preparation time:

10 minutes

Cooking time:

15 minutes

Standing time:

40 minutes

Canned lentils are easier to digest than dried.

TIP

The assembled salad can be covered and refrigerated for up to 2 days or frozen for up to 3 months. It reheats quite well in the microwave!

NUTRIENTS PER SERVING	
Calories	190
Protein	7 g
Fat	4.0 g
Saturated fat	0.5 g
Carbohydrates	33 g
Fiber	3 g
Sodium	140 mg

²/₃ cup	basmati rice	150 mL
1½ cups	water	375 mL
1 tbsp	extra virgin olive oil	15 mL
1½ tbsp	freshly squeezed lemon juice	22 mL
1 tbsp	soy sauce	15 mL
1 tsp	curry powder	5 mL
1 cup	rinsed drained canned lentils	250 mL
¼ cup	finely chopped fresh Italian (flat-leaf) parsley	60 mL
1 tsp	finely chopped fresh basil	5 mL
2 tbsp	finely chopped fresh chives	30 mL
	Freshly ground black pepper	

1. Place the rice in a fine-mesh strainer and hold it under cold running water until the water runs clear, then drain well.

2. Bring 1½ cups (375 mL) water to a boil in a saucepan. Add rice. Cover and cook over very low heat for about 15 minutes without uncovering. Remove saucepan from heat. The water should be completely absorbed. If it isn't, cover and simmer for a few more minutes. Let cool down for a few minutes, then let stand in the refrigerator for at least 30 minutes.

3. In a small bowl, combine the oil, lemon juice, soy sauce and curry powder.

4. Put the rice in a salad bowl. Add the lentils, parsley, basil and chives. Pour the vinaigrette over the salad, add a little ground pepper and toss gently. Let stand for 10 minutes, then serve.

Mixed Vegetable Salad with Eggs

Preparation time:

15 minutes

Cooking time:

20 minutes

2	potatoes (14 oz/400 g total)	2
4½ oz	green beans	130 g
2	large eggs	2
2	medium tomatoes	2
⅓ cup	Classic Vinaigrette (page 95)	75 mL
	Salt and freshly ground black pepper	
⅓	head curly leaf lettuce	⅓
12	black olives	12

1. Wash the potatoes and leave whole; do not peel. Place the potatoes in a steamer basket or in a pot of salted water to either steam or boil for 13 minutes.

2. Meanwhile, trim the ends of the green beans. Add the green beans to the potatoes and continue steaming or boiling for another 7 minutes, until the potatoes are tender and the beans are tender-crisp. Let the vegetables cool down for 10 minutes or longer, so they won't be so hot to handle. Cut the potatoes into slices and cut the beans into pieces.

3. Boil the eggs for 10 minutes, cool them down immediately in cold water, then peel and cut into quarters.

4. In a bowl, combine the potatoes, green beans and tomatoes. Pour on the Classic Vinaigrette, then season with salt and pepper to taste. Toss well.

5. Put the lettuce leaves in a salad bowl or on a serving plate and top with the potato mixture. Arrange the olives and quartered eggs on top of the salad and serve.

NUTRIENTS PER SERVING	
Calories	290
Protein	6 g
Fat	20.0 g
Saturated fat	3.0 g
Carbohydrates	22 g
Fiber	4 g
Sodium	190 mg

Soups and Sandwiches

Homemade Chicken Broth

• **MAKE AHEAD** •

• **FREEZABLE** •

Preparation time:

10 minutes

Cooking time:

1½ hours

Homemade chicken broth is a great comfort food with an excellent reputation as a remedy against colds and flu.

• **Large sieve or colander, lined with cheesecloth**

1	bulb fennel (12 oz/360 g)	1
3	whole cloves	3
2	carrots	2
2	stalks celery (5 oz/140 g total)	2
1	whole chicken (about 3 lbs/1.4 kg)	1
2	bay leaves	2
12 cups	water (approx.)	3 L
½ tsp	whole black peppercorns	2 mL
¾ tsp	salt (approx.)	3 mL
	Freshly ground black pepper	

1. Cut the fennel into quarters and stick the cloves into one of the quarters. Cut the carrots and celery stalks in half.

2. Place the fennel, carrots, celery, bay leaves and whole chicken (without the giblets!) into a pot. Add cold water to cover (2 to 2½ inches/5 to 6 cm above the chicken). Add peppercorns and salt (not too much, you can always add more later on).

3. Bring to a boil. Reduce to a very gentle simmer: liquid should just bubble up to the surface. Cook, uncovered, for 1 hour. A skin will form on the surface of the liquid; skim this off with a slotted or regular spoon and discard.

4. Remove the chicken and pick off the meat. Reserve the chicken meat in a tight container, covered with some of the broth, for another use. Let cool down for a few minutes, then put the container in the refrigerator.

TIPS

The FODMAP content of fennel and celery is borderline, so be sure to use the precise weights indicated in the recipe.

The broth keeps for up to 5 days in the refrigerator or up to 4 months in the freezer.

5. Adjust the seasoning of the broth with salt and pepper, then return the carcass to the pot. Simmer, uncovered, for another 30 minutes.

6. Remove from heat and, when the broth is cool enough to work with, strain it through a sieve or a colander lined with cheesecloth, discarding the carcass, herbs and vegetables. Transfer to an airtight container and refrigerate. Leave any remaining fat in the broth as a protective cover. You can skim it off when you use the broth.

Allergen-Free Vegetable Broth

**MAKES
8 CUPS (2 L)**

• MAKE AHEAD •

• FREEZABLE •

Preparation time:

10 minutes

Cooking time:

1 hour

Standing time:

30 minutes

*Use this broth in place
of ready-made broths
(which are full of onion
and garlic) in all recipes
that call for it.*

TIPS

The FODMAP content
of celery is borderline,
so be sure to use
the precise weight
indicated in the recipe.

The broth keeps for
up to 1 week in the
refrigerator or up to
4 months in the freezer.

• **Large sieve**

4	carrots (14 oz/400 g total)	4
4	stalks celery (9 oz/280 g total)	4
2	tomatoes	2
3 tbsp	olive oil	45 mL
1 tbsp	unseasoned pure tomato paste	15 mL
$\frac{1}{2}$	bunch fresh Italian (flat-leaf) parsley (1$\frac{1}{2}$ oz/50 g)	$\frac{1}{2}$
2	bay leaves	2
1 tsp	dried oregano	5 mL
1 tsp	coarse salt	5 mL
8 cups	water	2 L

1. Cut the carrots, celery and tomatoes in half. In a large pot, sweat carrots and celery in oil for 10 minutes, stirring from time to time.

2. Add the tomatoes, tomato paste, parsley, bay leaves, oregano, salt and water. Bring to a boil, then cover and simmer for 45 minutes. Let cool for about 30 minutes.

3. Strain broth through a sieve, pressing the vegetables to get the most broth. Discard solids.

Watercress Soup

MAKES 6 SERVINGS

• MAKE AHEAD •

• FREEZABLE •

Preparation time:

10 minutes

Cooking time:

20 minutes

TIP

The FODMAP content of fennel is borderline, so be sure to use the precise weight indicated in the recipe.

• **Blender**

2	bunches watercress (8 oz/240 g total)	2
1	small bulb fennel (8½ oz/260 g), trimmed	1
2	potatoes (14 oz/400 g total)	2
2 tbsp	non-hydrogenated margarine	30 mL
2 cups	Allergen-Free Vegetable Broth (page 116)	500 mL
2 cups	lactose-free milk	500 mL
	Salt and freshly ground black pepper	

1. Rinse the watercress carefully, without soaking it, to remove any sand. Chop most of it, reserving some leaves with stems for decoration. Coarsely chop the fennel. Peel and dice the potatoes into ½-inch (1 cm) cubes.

2. Heat the margarine in a saucepan over medium heat. Add the chopped fennel and sauté for 3 minutes, then add the potatoes and watercress. Continue to cook for about 4 minutes, stirring gently. Add the broth and lactose-free milk, bring to a boil, then lower the heat. Cover and simmer for about 15 minutes, until the vegetables are soft.

3. Purée the soup in the blender until smooth. Return the soup to the same saucepan and rewarm over low heat. Season to taste with salt and pepper.

4. Ladle the soup into bowls, garnish with the reserved watercress leaves and serve.

Vegan Variation

Oil may substitute for margarine and a low-FODMAP plant-based non-dairy milk may substitute for lactose-free milk.

NUTRIENTS PER SERVING

Calories	140
Protein	6 g
Fat	5.0 g
Saturated fat	1.0 g
Carbohydrates	20 g
Fiber	3 g
Sodium	200 mg

Spinach Soup

**MAKES
4 SERVINGS**

• **MAKE AHEAD** •

• **FREEZABLE** •

Preparation time:

5 minutes

Cooking time:

15 minutes

• **Blender**

6 cups	packed spinach, trimmed (6 oz/170 g)	1.5 L
	Salt	
1½ tbsp	non-hydrogenated margarine	22 mL
¼	bulb fennel (2⅔ oz/80 g)	¼
2 tbsp	white rice flour	30 mL
1¾ cups	lactose-free milk	375 mL
Pinch	grated nutmeg	Pinch
Pinch	cayenne pepper	Pinch
	Freshly ground black pepper	
2 tsp	slivered almonds	10 mL

1. Wash the spinach and drain it briefly, then transfer it to a pot or saucepan without adding any water. The water trapped in the leaves is enough to cook them. Add salt, then cover and cook over high heat for 3 to 4 minutes until the leaves wilt and turn a very deep green. Avoid overcooking; otherwise, the spinach will become brownish. Transfer the spinach to a colander, press to remove excess water and set aside.

2. While the spinach is cooking, heat the margarine in another saucepan over medium heat. Finely chop the fennel and add it to the saucepan. Sauté for 2 to 3 minutes, until it becomes translucent. Add the rice flour and cook for 1 minute, stirring. Gradually whisk in the milk. Bring the mixture to a boil, whisking constantly, and cook until it thickens, about 4 minutes. Remove the saucepan from the heat.

NUTRIENTS PER SERVING	
Calories	230
Protein	12 g
Fat	11.0 g
Saturated fat	2.5 g
Carbohydrates	22 g
Fiber	3 g
Sodium	180 mg

The FODMAP content
of fennel is borderline,
so be sure to use
the precise weight
indicated in the recipe.

The soup keeps for
up to 6 days in the
refrigerator or for up to
2 months in the freezer.

3. Add the spinach to the mixture. Let the mixture cool down for a few minutes, then purée it in a blender. Return the soup to the same saucepan and rewarm over low heat. Season with the grated nutmeg, cayenne pepper, salt and pepper to taste.

4. Ladle the soup into bowls, sprinkle with the sliced almonds and serve.

Vegan Variation

Oil may substitute for margarine and unsweetened almond milk or soy milk (from soy protein) may substitute for lactose-free milk.

Carrot and Mint Soup [VEGAN OPTION]

Preparation time:

10 minutes

Cooking time:

20 minutes

TIP

The soup keeps for up to 7 days in the refrigerator or up to 4 months in the freezer.

• **Blender**

4	carrots (14 oz/400 g total)	4
1 tbsp	Garlic-Infused Oil (page 147)	15 mL
1²⁄₃ cups	Allergen-Free Vegetable Broth (page 116)	400 mL
1¹⁄₂ cups	lactose-free milk	375 mL
2¹⁄₂ tbsp	chopped fresh mint	37 mL
2 tbsp	chopped fresh chives	30 mL
8	drops hot pepper sauce, such as Tabasco	8
	Salt and freshly ground black pepper	
	Fresh mint leaves	

1. Peel carrots and cut into 1¹⁄₄-inch (3 cm) pieces.

2. Heat the Garlic-Infused Oil in a saucepan over medium heat. Add the carrots and cook for 5 minutes, with occasional stirring. Add the broth and lactose-free milk; bring to a boil, then lower the heat. Cover and simmer for about 15 minutes, until the vegetables are soft.

3. Purée the soup in the blender until smooth. Return the soup to the same saucepan and rewarm over low heat. Add the chopped mint, chives and hot pepper sauce, and season to taste with salt and pepper.

4. Ladle the soup into bowls, garnish with fresh mint leaves and serve.

> **Vegan Variation**
>
> Plain almond milk or soy milk (from soy protein) may be substituted for lactose-free milk.

NUTRIENTS PER SERVING

Calories	130
Protein	5 g
Fat	5.0 g
Saturated fat	1.0 g
Carbohydrates	16 g
Fiber	4 g
Sodium	260 mg

Carrot Soup with Orange and Ginger

**MAKES
4 SERVINGS**

· **MAKE AHEAD** ·

· **FREEZABLE** ·

Preparation time:

10 minutes

Cooking time:

30 minutes

TIPS

The FODMAP content of fennel is borderline, so be sure to use the precise weight indicated in the recipe.

The soup keeps for up to 7 days in the refrigerator or up to 4 months in the freezer.

NUTRIENTS PER SERVING	
Calories	170
Protein	3 g
Fat	7.0 g
Saturated fat	1.0 g
Carbohydrates	28 g
Fiber	7 g
Sodium	460 mg

- **Blender**

1 tbsp	canola oil	15 mL
½	bulb fennel (6 oz/170 g), coarsely chopped	½
6	carrots (1¼ lbs/600 g total), coarsely chopped	6
⅔ cup	unsweetened orange juice	175 mL
2½ tbsp	coarsely grated gingerroot	37 mL
4 cups	Allergen-Free Vegetable Broth (page 116)	1 L
	Salt and freshly ground black pepper	

1. Heat oil in a pot over medium heat. Sweat the fennel for about 3 to 4 minutes, stirring often. Add the carrots, orange juice, ginger and broth. Bring to a boil, then lower the heat, cover and simmer until the carrots are tender, about 25 minutes.

2. Purée the soup in the blender, then pour it back into the pot and warm it up for a few minutes. Adjust the seasoning with salt and pepper, then serve.

Silky Smooth Roasted Pepper Soup

**MAKES
4 SERVINGS**

· MAKE AHEAD ·

· FREEZABLE ·

Preparation time:

10 minutes

Cooking time:

30 minutes

TIPS

The FODMAP content of fennel is borderline, so be sure to use the precise weight indicated in the recipe.

The soup keeps for up to 7 days in the refrigerator or up to 4 months in the freezer.

NUTRIENTS PER SERVING

Calories	220
Protein	3 g
Fat	12.0 g
Saturated fat	1.5 g
Carbohydrates	28 g
Fiber	5 g
Sodium	300 mg

- Preheat oven to 400°F (200°C)
- Baking sheet, oiled
- Blender

2	potatoes (14 oz/400 g total)	2
3 cups	Allergen-Free Vegetable Broth (page 116)	750 mL
2	yellow or red bell peppers	2
1½ tsp	Garlic-Infused Oil (page 147)	7 mL
½	bulb fennel (6 oz/170 g), trimmed and finely chopped	½
	Salt and freshly ground black pepper	

1. Peel the potatoes and put them in a pot. Pour in the broth. Bring to a boil, then lower the heat and simmer until the potatoes are soft, about 15 minutes.

2. Meanwhile, cut the bell peppers in half, removing the seeds, cores and stems, then put them, cut side down, on prepared baking sheet. Roast in the middle of the preheated oven until they are soft, about 15 minutes. Turn them once halfway through cooking. (Alternatively, grill the peppers on an outdoor grill.)

3. Remove the peppers from the oven, cover them and let them cool down for about 10 minutes.

4. Meanwhile, heat the Garlic-Infused Oil in a heavy frying pan over medium heat. Add the fennel and cook, stirring, until softened, about 5 minutes. Peel the peppers, add them to the pan and cook for 5 minutes. Add the vegetable mixture to the pot of broth. Cook for a couple of minutes. Add salt and pepper to taste.

5. Purée the soup in the blender until a creamy consistency is obtained. Return the soup to the same pot and rewarm over low heat. Serve.

My Grandma's Cream of Tomato Soup

VEGAN

Preparation time:

5 minutes

Cooking time:

15 minutes

Many studies have shown that consumption of fresh or processed tomatoes is linked to a reduction in the risk of certain cancers, especially prostate.

TIP

The soup keeps for up to 7 days in the refrigerator or up to 4 months in the freezer.

NUTRIENTS PER SERVING	
Calories	130
Protein	1 g
Fat	7.0 g
Saturated fat	0.5 g
Carbohydrates	15 g
Fiber	2 g
Sodium	320 mg

3½ tbsp	canola oil	52 mL
6 tbsp	cornstarch	90 mL
3 cups	lukewarm Allergen-Free Vegetable Broth (page 116; approx.)	750 mL
2½ cups	tomato passata (see tip, page 188)	625 mL
	Salt and freshly ground black pepper	
	Hot pepper sauce, such as Tabasco	

1. Heat the oil in a saucepan over low heat. Add the cornstarch and beat well with a whisk or wooden spoon. Cook for 3 minutes, stirring constantly and taking care not to let it burn. Slowly add 3 cups (750 mL) broth, stirring thoroughly to avoid lumps. Cook over medium heat for 4 to 5 minutes.

2. Add the tomatoes and mix well. Add more broth if the soup is too thick. Cook for 5 minutes over medium heat. Season with salt, pepper and hot pepper sauce to taste, then serve.

Root Vegetable Soup with Dill

**MAKES
6 SERVINGS**

· MAKE AHEAD ·

Preparation time:

15 minutes

Cooking time:

30 minutes

*This is a traditional
Russian soup. Earthy
root vegetables, cooked
with fresh spinach, are
enlivened here with a
tart, fresh topping of
dill and lemon.*

TIP

The soup keeps for
up to 7 days in the
refrigerator; store
cooked eggs in the
shell separately and
peel just before serving.

NUTRIENTS PER SERVING

Calories	210
Protein	8 g
Fat	6.0 g
Saturated fat	1.5 g
Carbohydrates	32 g
Fiber	7 g
Sodium	440 mg

2	potatoes (14 oz/400 g total)	2
2	carrots	2
1	large turnip (8½ oz/260 g)	1
1	parsnip	1
1	small bulb fennel (8½ oz/260 g) (see tip, page 127)	1
½	celeriac (11 oz/320 g)	½
5 cups	Allergen-Free Vegetable Broth (page 116)	1.25 L
3	large eggs	3
9 cups	lightly packed spinach (8 oz/240 g), trimmed	2.25 L
	Salt and freshly ground black pepper	
½ cup	fresh dill	125 mL
1	lemon, cut into quarters	1

1. Peel the potatoes, carrots, turnips, parsnips, fennel and celeriac, then cut them into uniform 1-inch (2.5 cm) pieces.

2. Put all the vegetables and broth into a pot. Bring to a boil, then reduce the heat, cover and simmer until the vegetables are tender, about 25 minutes.

3. Meanwhile, place the eggs in a saucepan of cold water. Bring to a boil, then remove from the heat and let stand for 15 minutes. Cool them down immediately in cold water, then cut them into halves. Set aside.

4. Add the spinach to the soup and cook until it is wilted, about 2 to 3 minutes. Season with salt and pepper to taste. Finely chop the dill and add it to the soup.

5. Ladle the soup into bowls. Garnish each bowl with half a boiled egg, along with lemon quarters. Serve.

Winter Vegetable Soup VEGAN

Preparation time:

10 minutes

Cooking time:

30 minutes

TIPS

The FODMAP content of celery and fennel is borderline, so be sure to use the precise weights indicated in the recipe.

The soup keeps for up to 7 days in the refrigerator or up to 4 months in the freezer.

• **Blender**

3	potatoes (1¼ lbs/600 g total)	3
3	parsnips	3
2	carrots	2
2	turnips	2
3	stalks celery (7 oz/220 g total)	3
1	bulb fennel (11 oz/340 g), trimmed	1
2 tbsp	olive oil	30 mL
	Salt and freshly ground black pepper	
	Cayenne pepper (optional)	
5 cups	warm Allergen-Free Vegetable Broth (page 116)	1.25 L

1. Peel the potatoes, parsnips, carrots and turnips. Coarsely cut all the vegetables into uniform 1¼-inch (3 cm) pieces.

2. Heat the oil in a saucepan over medium heat. Add all the vegetables and cook over medium heat for about 10 minutes, stirring occasionally. Season with salt, pepper and a pinch of cayenne pepper, if desired.

3. Pour in the warm broth. Cook, uncovered, until the potatoes are cooked and fork-tender, about 20 minutes.

4. Purée the soup in the blender. Return the soup to the same saucepan and rewarm over low heat. Adjust the seasoning. Serve.

NUTRIENTS PER SERVING

Calories	170
Protein	3 g
Fat	5.0 g
Saturated fat	0.5 g
Carbohydrates	30 g
Fiber	6 g
Sodium	300 mg

Parsnip and Potato Soup

Preparation time:

10 minutes

Cooking time:

30 minutes

TIPS

The FODMAP content of celery and fennel is borderline, so be sure to use the precise weights indicated in the recipe.

The soup keeps for up to 7 days in the refrigerator or up to 4 months in the freezer.

NUTRIENTS PER SERVING	
Calories	170
Protein	5 g
Fat	6.0 g
Saturated fat	2.0 g
Carbohydrates	27 g
Fiber	5 g
Sodium	300 mg

• **Blender**

4	parsnips (13 oz/380 g total)	4
2	potatoes (14 oz/400 g total), peeled	2
1	stalk celery (2⅓ oz/70 g)	1
½	bulb fennel (6½ oz/180 g)	½
1 tbsp	olive oil	15 mL
3 cups	warm Allergen-Free Vegetable Broth (page 116)	750 mL
	Salt and freshly ground black pepper	
½ cup	lactose-free milk	125 mL
1½ oz	feta cheese, crumbled	45 g
1 tbsp	finely chopped fresh chives	15 mL

1. Cut the parsnips, potatoes, celery and fennel into uniform 1¼-inch (3 cm) pieces.

2. Heat the oil in a saucepan over medium heat. Add all the vegetables and cook over medium heat for about 10 minutes, stirring occasionally.

3. Pour in the warm broth. Cook, uncovered, until the potatoes are fork-tender, about 15 to 20 minutes.

4. Purée the soup in the blender, then pour it back into the pot. Adjust the seasoning with salt and pepper, then add lactose-free milk and reheat.

5. Ladle soup into bowls, sprinkle with feta cheese and chives, then serve.

Vegan Variation

A low-FODMAP plant-based non-dairy milk may substitute for lactose-free milk. You can omit the feta cheese or replace it with some soft tofu.

Rice and Lentil Soup

VEGAN

Preparation time:

15 minutes

Cooking time:

35 minutes

TIPS

The FODMAP content of fennel is borderline, so be sure to use the precise weight indicated in the recipe.

The soup keeps for up to 7 days in the refrigerator or up to 3 months in the freezer.

1	bulb fennel (12 oz/360 g), trimmed	1
2	carrots	2
3 cups	packed Swiss chard or spinach, trimmed	750 mL
1½ tbsp	Garlic-Infused Oil (page 147)	22 mL
1 tsp	ground cumin	5 mL
6 cups	Allergen-Free Vegetable Broth (page 116)	1.5 L
½ cup	Arborio rice	125 mL
1¼ cups	canned diced tomatoes, with juice	300 mL
⅓ cup	drained rinsed canned lentils	75 mL
	Salt and freshly ground black pepper	

1. Finely chop the fennel and carrots. Coarsely chop the Swiss chard (green and white parts). Set aside.

2. Heat the Garlic-Infused Oil in a large pot over medium heat. Add the fennel and carrots, then cook for 5 minutes, stirring occasionally, until they are softened and lightly colored. Add the cumin and stir for 1 minute.

3. Pour in the broth, rice, tomatoes and lentils. Bring to a boil, then reduce the heat, cover and simmer until the rice is cooked, about 25 minutes.

4. Add the chard to the soup, cover and simmer until the chard is tender, about 5 minutes. Season with salt and pepper to taste. Thin the soup with more broth or water, if desired, then serve.

NUTRIENTS PER SERVING	
Calories	140
Protein	4 g
Fat	5.0 g
Saturated fat	0.5 g
Carbohydrates	22 g
Fiber	5 g
Sodium	430 mg

Fresh Mozzarella and Tomato Sandwich

Preparation time:

5 minutes

TIP
You may try 100% spelt sourdough bread in this recipe. Even though spelt does contain FODMAPs (fructans), the long fermentation of the sourdough bread breaks down most of them, making this bread a great alternative to wheat-free.

2	slices gluten-free bread (3 oz/ 90 g total)	2
1	tomato, cut into slices	1
1	ball bocconcini (fresh mozzarella), cut into slices (2 oz/55 g)	1
½ tsp	extra virgin olive oil	2 mL
½ tsp	dried oregano	2 mL
	Salt and freshly ground black pepper	

1. Top 1 slice of bread with tomato and bocconcini slices, then drizzle with oil and sprinkle with oregano. Season with salt and pepper, then sandwich with the other bread slice. Serve.

NUTRIENTS PER SERVING	
Calories	340
Protein	15 g
Fat	18.0 g
Saturated fat	8.0 g
Carbohydrates	33 g
Fiber	6 g
Sodium	300 mg

Tofu Salad Wrap

VEGAN

Preparation time:

10 minutes

Standing time:

30 minutes

TIP

It's important to remove as much water as possible from the tofu, to allow it to absorb flavor. To do so, either drain well or freeze the tofu block in a plastic bag, then thaw in a sieve over a bowl in the fridge before using it.

3½ oz	firm regular tofu (see tip)	100 g
1 tbsp	canola oil	15 mL
1 tbsp	freshly squeezed lemon juice	15 mL
¾ tsp	nutritional yeast	3 mL
2 tsp	Dijon mustard	10 mL
⅛ tsp	cayenne pepper	0.5 mL
⅛ tsp	ground turmeric	0.5 mL
1½ tsp	finely chopped fresh Italian (flat-leaf) parsley	7 mL
¾ tsp	finely chopped fresh dill	3 mL
1	green onion (green part only), chopped	1
1	6-inch (15 cm) corn tortilla	1
¼ cup	packed baby spinach	60 mL

1. Crumble the tofu into a bowl. Add the oil, lemon juice, nutritional yeast, mustard, cayenne, turmeric, parsley, dill and green onion, mixing well. Let rest in the refrigerator for at least 30 minutes, to let the flavors develop.

2. Place the tortilla on a work surface. Spread tofu mixture onto tortilla. Add spinach, roll tortilla into a wrap and serve.

NUTRIENTS PER SERVING	
Calories	370
Protein	19 g
Fat	23.0 g
Saturated fat	2.1 g
Carbohydrates	27 g
Fiber	4 g
Sodium	170 mg

Egg Salad Sandwich

Preparation time:

5 minutes

Although celery is often identified as a high-FODMAP food, in small quantities, as in this recipe, it is usually well tolerated.

TIP

The FODMAP content of celery is borderline, so be sure to use the precise weight indicated in the recipe.

1	large egg, hard boiled, chopped	1
½ tsp	finely chopped fresh chives	2 mL
½	stalk celery (1 oz/35 g), finely chopped	½
1 tsp	mayonnaise	5 mL
	Salt and freshly ground black pepper	
2	slices gluten-free bread (3 oz/ 90 g total)	2
¼ cup	packed baby spinach or 1 lettuce leaf	60 mL

1. Combine egg, chives, celery and mayonnaise in a bowl; season with salt and pepper.
2. Spread egg mixture on 1 slice of bread, top with spinach, then sandwich with the other bread slice. Serve.

NUTRIENTS PER SERVING

Calories	290
Protein	12 g
Fat	14.0 g
Saturated fat	3.0 g
Carbohydrates	31 g
Fiber	5 g
Sodium	350 mg

Pan Bagnat

MAKES 2 SERVINGS

Preparation time:

15 minutes

Standing time:

4 hours

Pan bagnat used to be a staple food of fishermen in Provence, France. Its name means "wet bread" in the local dialect and refers to bread that has been soaked in olive oil. It is still a very popular lunch in Nice and Côte d'Azur.

2	gluten-free ciabatta-style panini rolls (6 oz/180 g total)	2
4 tsp	Garlic-Infused Oil (page 147)	20 mL
¼	bunch arugula	¼
1 tbsp	Classic Vinaigrette (page 95)	15 mL
½	green onion (green part only), finely chopped	½
	Salt and freshly ground black pepper	
1	tomato, thinly sliced	1
1	large egg, hard-cooked and sliced	1
4	black olives, pitted	4
1	can (6 oz/170 g) tuna, drained	1
4	leaves fresh basil (optional)	4
1	radish, thinly sliced	1

1. Slice each panini roll lengthwise into 2 halves and baste the cut sides with the Garlic-Infused Oil.

2. Put the arugula in a bowl. Pour in the Classic Vinaigrette and add the green onion. Season with salt and pepper to taste, then mix well.

3. Portion out the arugula mixture onto bottom halves of rolls. Distribute the tomato slices, hard-cooked egg, olives, tuna and radish slices on top of the arugula. Garnish with the basil leaves (if using). Cover with the top halves of rolls.

4. Wrap each sandwich individually with plastic wrap, then chill under a weight in the refrigerator for a minimum of 4 hours and a maximum of 12 hours. Enjoy.

NUTRIENTS PER SERVING	
Calories	480
Protein	30 g
Fat	27.0 g
Saturated fat	4.5 g
Carbohydrates	33 g
Fiber	6 g
Sodium	390 mg

Lobster Roll

**MAKES
1 SERVING**

• MAKE AHEAD •

Preparation time:

10 minutes

Cooking time:

10 minutes

This is a staple summer meal throughout New England and the Maritime provinces of Canada, with plenty of variations, depending on the location and the restaurant. Now you can create your own!

1	live lobster (about 1 lb/500 g)	1
2 tsp	freshly squeezed lemon juice	10 mL
2 tsp	mayonnaise	10 mL
1 tsp	ketchup	5 mL
$\frac{1}{4}$	stalk celery ($\frac{1}{2}$ oz/18 g), thinly sliced	$\frac{1}{4}$
$\frac{1}{2}$	radish, thinly sliced	$\frac{1}{2}$
1	gluten-free roll or bun (3 oz/90 g), split in half, or 2 slices gluten-free bread (3 oz/90 g total)	1
2 tbsp	mixed salad greens	30 mL
	Salt and freshly ground black pepper	

1. Remove the elastic bands from the claws and plunge the lobster, head first, into a large pot of salted boiling water, with the tail tucked underneath (to avoid being splashed by the tail). Loosely cover the pot and cook the lobster over medium-high heat until the shell turns red, about 5 minutes from the time the water comes to a boil again. Using tongs, transfer the lobster to a sink to drain and cool.

2. When the lobster is cool enough to handle, twist off the claws and crack them, then remove the meat. Halve the lobster lengthwise with a large knife or poultry shears, beginning from the tail end, then remove the tail meat. Cut all the lobster meat into bite-size pieces, then set aside.

NUTRIENTS PER SERVING

Calories	350
Protein	27 g
Fat	13.0 g
Saturated fat	2.0 g
Carbohydrates	34 g
Fiber	5 g
Sodium	690 g

TIPS

The FODMAP content of celery is borderline, so be sure to use the precise weight indicated in the recipe.

You can start with a cooked lobster and skip step 1.

The lobster can be cooked and shelled ahead and stored in the refrigerator for up to 1 day. The lobster filling can be prepared and kept in the refrigerator for up to 1 day.

3. In a bowl, stir together the lemon juice, mayonnaise and ketchup until well blended. Mix in the celery and radish. Lightly mix in the lobster so it just gets coated without falling apart.

4. Spread the lobster filling on the bottom half of the roll or bun (or on 1 slice of bread), top with greens, then season with salt and pepper. Sandwich with the top half of the roll or bun (or the other bread slice), then enjoy.

Turkey and Cheese Sandwich

Preparation time:

5 minutes

Did you know that radishes are part of the cruciferous family, just like broccoli? Due to their vitamin, mineral and antioxidant content, radishes can play a role in the prevention of certain cancers and cardiovascular diseases, as well as being low in FODMAPs!

2	slices gluten-free bread (3 oz/ 90 g total)	2
1	slice roasted turkey breast ($^2/_3$ oz/20 g)	1
1	slice low-fat cheese ($^2/_3$ oz/22 g)	1
$^1/_4$ cup	packed baby spinach (or 1 lettuce leaf)	60 mL
1	radish, thinly sliced	1

1. Top 1 slice of bread with turkey, cheese, spinach and radish slices, then sandwich with the other bread slice. Serve.

NUTRIENTS PER SERVING

Calories	240
Protein	14 g
Fat	7.0 g
Saturated fat	2.0 g
Carbohydrates	31 g
Fiber	5 g
Sodium	560 mg

Ham and Cheese Sandwich

Preparation time:

5 minutes

TIP

Be careful to choose a ham without any flavorings, in particular no garlic or onion powders, which are high in FODMAPs.

2	slices gluten-free bread (3 oz/90 g total)	2
½ tsp	Dijon mustard	2 mL
1	slice ham (⅔ oz/20 g)	1
1	slice low-fat cheese (⅔ oz/22 g)	1
¼ cup	packed baby spinach or 1 lettuce leaf	60 mL

1. Spread 1 slice of bread with mustard, then top with ham, cheese and spinach. Sandwich with the other bread slice. Serve.

NUTRIENTS PER SERVING

Calories	230
Protein	14 g
Fat	7.0 g
Saturated fat	2.0 g
Carbohydrates	30 g
Fiber	5 g
Sodium	580 mg

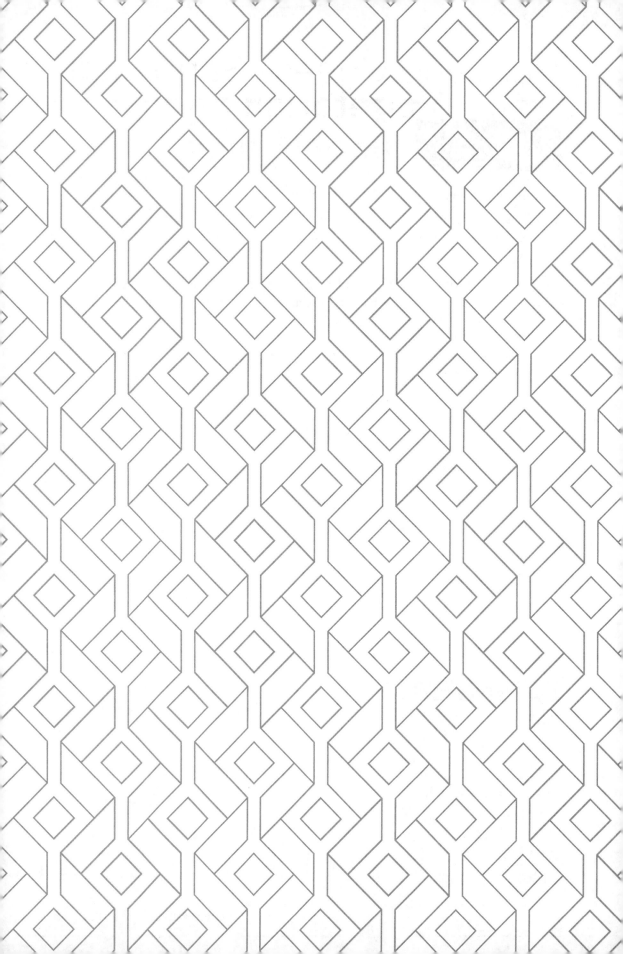

Vegetarian and Vegan Mains

Warm Quinoa and Arugula Salad

MAKES 4 SERVINGS

• **MAKE AHEAD** •

Preparation time:

10 minutes

Cooking time:

15 minutes

Aromatic herbs, like mint, are low-FODMAP. Don't hesitate to add them to your recipes to add flavor when you're eliminating garlic and onion.

TIP

The salad, without the arugula, can be prepared, covered and refrigerated for up to 1 day. Add the arugula just before serving.

NUTRIENTS PER SERVING	
Calories	360
Protein	14 g
Fat	18.0 g
Saturated fat	4.0 g
Carbohydrates	38 g
Fiber	4 g
Sodium	590 mg

1⅔ cups	quinoa	400 mL
3 cups	water	750 mL
	Salt	
1	large bunch arugula (7 oz/200 g)	1
6 tbsp	chopped fresh mint	90 mL
3 tbsp	extra virgin olive oil	45 mL
4 tsp	freshly squeezed lemon juice	20 mL
	Freshly ground black pepper	
4 oz	light feta cheese, cut into small cubes	120 g

1. Place the quinoa in a fine-mesh strainer and hold it under cold running water until the water runs clear, then drain well.

2. Combine the quinoa, water and a pinch of salt in a saucepan. Bring to a boil, then reduce to a simmer. Cover and cook until the grains are translucent and the germ has spiraled out from each grain, about 15 minutes.

3. Meanwhile, clean the arugula and add it and the mint to a salad bowl.

4. Pour the oil and lemon juice into a small bowl, add salt and pepper to taste, and beat with a fork until the mixture is well combined.

5. Add the quinoa to the salad bowl. Pour the dressing over the salad and toss well. Add the feta cheese, adjust the seasoning and serve.

Quinoa and Pecan Salad

· MAKE AHEAD ·

Preparation time:

10 minutes

Cooking time:

15 minutes

Standing time:

2 hours

Although most nuts and seeds do contain some FODMAPs, they have plenty of great nutrition to offer and should be added in small quantities to your diet.

1 cup	quinoa	250 mL
2 cups	water	500 mL
	Salt	
3/4 cup	pecans, coarsely chopped	175 mL
3 tbsp	dried cranberries	45 mL
3	sprigs fresh thyme, leaves finely chopped	3
	Grated zest and juice of 1 orange	
3 tbsp	canola oil	45 mL
2 tsp	balsamic vinegar	10 mL
2 3/4 oz	light feta cheese, crumbled	80 g

1. Place the quinoa in a fine-mesh strainer and hold it under cold running water until the water runs clear, then drain well.

2. Combine the quinoa, water and a pinch of salt in a saucepan. Bring to a boil, then reduce to a simmer. Cover and cook until the grains are translucent and the germ has spiraled out from each grain, about 15 minutes. Transfer the quinoa to a bowl and let it cool down for about 1 hour at room temperature.

3. Add the pecans, cranberries, thyme, orange zest, orange juice, oil, vinegar, feta cheese and salt to taste. Mix well.

4. Chill in the refrigerator for about 1 hour to allow the flavors to meld. Adjust the seasoning and serve.

NUTRIENTS PER SERVING	
Calories	370
Protein	10 g
Fat	22.0 g
Saturated fat	3.0 g
Carbohydrates	34 g
Fiber	4 g
Sodium	390 mg

Asian Vegetable Soup VEGAN

**MAKES
4 SERVINGS**

Preparation time:

10 minutes

Cooking time:

10 minutes

*A hearty soup that's a
meal in itself.*

3 tbsp	soy sauce	45 mL
1½ tsp	sesame oil	7 mL
14 oz	firm regular tofu	400 g
5½ oz	rice stick noodles	160 g
2	carrots, grated	2
1 cup	thinly sliced savoy cabbage	250 mL
6 cups	Allergen-Free Vegetable Broth (page 116)	1.5 L
2 tsp	grated gingerroot	10 mL
1	dried chile pepper, minced	1
4 tsp	canola oil	20 mL
¼ cup	freshly squeezed lime juice	60 mL
3 tbsp	fresh cilantro leaves (optional)	45 mL

1. In a shallow dish, mix the soy sauce and sesame oil. Cut the tofu into ¾-inch (2 cm) cubes and add them to the marinade. Mix well, then let stand at room temperature while preparing the rest of the soup.

2. Meanwhile, cook the rice sticks in a large pot of boiling water according to package directions; drain and set aside.

3. Portion out the carrots and cabbage into 4 individual bowls.

4. Heat the broth in a saucepan. Add the ginger and chile pepper. Cook for 2 minutes.

5. Heat the canola oil in a skillet over medium heat. Add the tofu cubes and sauté for 3 to 4 minutes, with occasional stirring, until they are golden brown.

6. Pour the hot broth into the bowls. Add the tofu, rice sticks and lime juice. Garnish the bowls with whole cilantro leaves (if using) and serve.

NUTRIENTS PER SERVING

Calories	430
Protein	18 g
Fat	17.0 g
Saturated fat	2.0 g
Carbohydrates	54 g
Fiber	6 g
Sodium	780 mg

Fusilli with Watercress and Feta Cheese

Preparation time:

10 minutes

Cooking time:

15 minutes

TIP

Keep the serving plates in the oven at the lowest setting so they are warm when you serve.

2¾ oz	feta cheese	80 g
3 tbsp	chopped fresh dill	45 mL
3 tbsp	freshly squeezed lemon juice	45 mL
1	bunch watercress (2¾ oz/80 g)	1
11 oz	gluten-free (or wheat-free) fusilli (5 cups/1.25 L)	320 g
3 tbsp	olive oil	45 mL
12	black olives	12
	Freshly ground black pepper	

1. In a bowl, coarsely crumble the feta cheese and combine it with the chopped dill. Pour in the lemon juice, mix well, then set aside to marinate for about 10 minutes.

2. Rinse the watercress carefully, without soaking it, to remove any sand. Remove any thick stems and set aside.

3. Meanwhile, cook the fusilli in a large pot of salted boiling water until al dente. Drain.

4. Heat the oil in a pan over medium-low heat. Add the feta mixture and the olives, then cook for a few minutes. Add the watercress to the pan (keeping a few leaves with some stems for decoration) and heat for just 1 to 2 more minutes. It is important not to leave the watercress on the heat for too long, to avoid excessive wilting.

5. Pour the drained pasta into the pan. Mix well and add pepper to taste. Serve in warmed dishes. Garnish with the reserved watercress leaves.

NUTRIENTS PER SERVING	
Calories	430
Protein	11 g
Fat	15.0 g
Saturated fat	4.5 g
Carbohydrates	62 g
Fiber	3 g
Sodium	370 mg

Tofu Burgers

**MAKES
4 SERVINGS**

• **MAKE AHEAD** •

• **FREEZABLE** •

Preparation time:

15 minutes

Cooking time:

30 minutes

• **Preheat oven to 350°F (180°C)**
• **Food processor**
• **Baking sheet, lined with parchment paper**

²⁄₃ cup	long-grain brown or white rice	150 mL
9 oz	firm regular tofu, cut into chunks	260 g
½ cup	coarsely chopped fresh chives	125 mL
1 cup	coarsely chopped fresh Italian (flat-leaf) parsley (2¾ oz/80 g)	250 mL
2 tbsp	soy sauce	30 mL
2 tsp	paprika	10 mL
8	drops hot pepper sauce, such as Tabasco	8
	Salt and freshly ground black pepper	
2	large eggs, beaten	2
3 tbsp	canola oil	45 mL
4	slices gluten-free bread (6 oz/ 180 g total)	4
2 tbsp	mayonnaise	30 mL

1. Cook the rice according to package directions, then let it cool down for a few minutes.

2. In the food processor, combine the rice, tofu, chives, parsley, soy sauce, paprika and hot pepper sauce, then pulse until coarsely ground. Adjust the seasoning with salt and pepper.

3. Transfer to a bowl and stir in the beaten eggs. Shape the dough into 4 large patties or 8 small ones.

4. Heat the oil in a pan over medium-high heat. Cook the patties on one side for about 4 minutes, until golden, then gently flip and cook on the other side for about 5 minutes.

NUTRIENTS PER SERVING

Calories	450
Protein	19 g
Fat	23.0 g
Saturated fat	3.0 g
Carbohydrates	43 g
Fiber	4 g
Sodium	470 mg

Uncooked burger patties can be stored in airtight containers in the refrigerator for up to 2 days or frozen for up to 2 months. Let thaw in refrigerator overnight before cooking. Cook as directed, increasing baking time if necessary. Leftover cooked patties can be wrapped and refrigerated for up to 2 days.

5. Transfer the patties to the prepared baking sheet and bake in the middle of the preheated oven for about 30 minutes or until they are firm and cooked through on the inside.

6. Serve the patties on bread and top with a spoonful of mayonnaise.

Vegan Variation

Replace the eggs with 2 tbsp (30 mL) ground flax seeds (flaxseed meal) mixed with $\frac{2}{3}$ cup (150 mL) water. Let stand for 5 minutes before adding to the recipe, to allow it to gel. Omit the mayonnaise or replace it with a low-FODMAP vegan condiment.

Vegetable Fritters

**MAKES
4 SERVINGS**

• **MAKE AHEAD** •

• **FREEZABLE** •

Preparation time:

10 minutes

Cooking time:

25 minutes

TIPS

The FODMAP content of sweet potato is borderline, so be sure to use the precise weight indicated.

These fritters may be kept in airtight containers in the refrigerator for up to 2 days or for up to 3 to 4 weeks in the freezer. Warm thawed fritters in a 400°F (200°C) oven for about 10 minutes.

NUTRIENTS PER SERVING	
Calories	210
Protein	10 g
Fat	11.0 g
Saturated fat	3.5 g
Carbohydrates	18 g
Fiber	4 g
Sodium	300 mg

• **Preheat oven to 400°F (200°C)**
• **1 or 2 large baking sheets, lined with parchment paper**

3	carrots (10 oz/300 g total)	3
2	zucchini (9 oz/260 g total)	2
1	large sweet potato (8½ oz/240 g), peeled	1
⅔ cup	grated Parmesan cheese (1¾ oz/50 g)	150 mL
2	large eggs, beaten	2
1½ tbsp	olive oil	22 mL
⅛ tsp	cayenne pepper	0.5 mL
Pinch	salt	Pinch
	Freshly ground black pepper	

1. Coarsely grate the carrots, zucchini and sweet potato. Put all the vegetables in a bowl and stir in the cheese. Add the eggs, oil, cayenne pepper and a little salt and pepper to taste. Mix well, then portion out the mixture onto the prepared baking sheet(s), forming 14 to 16 rounds about 4 inches (10 cm) in diameter.

2. Bake in the middle of the preheated oven for 12 minutes, then delicately turn over the fritters and continue to cook until they are golden-colored, about 12 more minutes. Serve.

Baked Tofu with Ginger

VEGAN

**MAKES
4 SERVINGS**

Preparation time:

10 minutes

Marinating time:

20 minutes

Cooking time:

15 minutes

TIP

Unless you suffer from celiac disease or gluten intolerance, it is not necessary to choose a gluten-free soy sauce. The traces of wheat that may be found in regular soy sauce are not enough to cause symptoms.

- **Preheat oven to 400°F (200°C)**

1¼ lbs	firm regular tofu	600 g
3 tbsp	soy sauce	45 mL
1½ tbsp	canola oil	22 mL
4 tsp	unseasoned rice vinegar	20 mL
1½ tsp	sesame oil	7 mL
4 tsp	chopped fresh Italian (flat-leaf) parsley	20 mL
4 tsp	grated gingerroot	20 mL

1. Cut the tofu into ⅔-inch (1.5 cm) thick slices. Arrange the slices in a single layer in a baking dish.

2. Combine the soy sauce, canola oil, rice vinegar, sesame oil, parsley and ginger in a bowl. Mix well and pour the marinade over the tofu. Marinate at room temperature for about 20 minutes.

3. Bake the tofu in the marinade in the preheated oven for 12 to 15 minutes. If tofu is too dry, add a small amount of water. Serve.

NUTRIENTS PER SERVING	
Calories	230
Protein	21 g
Fat	15.0 g
Saturated fat	1.5 g
Carbohydrates	5 g
Fiber	0 g
Sodium	150 mg

Indian-Style Tofu Sauté VEGAN

Preparation time:

10 minutes

Cooking time:

25 minutes

An example of "China meets India" in a hurry: a quick sauté in a wok followed by Indian curry seasoning.

TIPS

The FODMAP content of fennel is borderline, so be sure to use the precise weight indicated in the recipe.

This dish can be cooled and stored in an airtight container in the refrigerator for up to 3 days.

NUTRIENTS PER SERVING

Calories	330
Protein	21 g
Fat	24.0 g
Saturated fat	6.0 g
Carbohydrates	13 g
Fiber	3 g
Sodium	55 mg

• **Preheat oven to 170°F (77°C)**

¼ cup	Garlic-Infused Oil (opposite), divided	60 mL
14 oz	firm regular tofu, diced	400 g
½	bulb fennel (6 oz/170 g), trimmed and finely chopped	½
2	zucchini (9 oz/260 g total), cut into rounds	2
1	green bell pepper, cut into thin strips	1
1 tbsp	curry powder, divided	15 mL
2 cups	bean sprouts	500 mL
	Salt	
⅔ cup	light unsweetened coconut milk	150 mL
	Freshly ground black pepper	

1. Heat 1 tbsp (15 mL) Garlic-Infused Oil in a skillet or wok over medium heat. Sauté the tofu for 7 to 8 minutes, until it is golden-colored, stirring gently from time to time. Remove the tofu from the skillet, place in a dish and keep warm in the oven.

2. Add 1 tbsp (15 mL) Garlic-Infused Oil to the skillet over medium heat and sauté the fennel. Add the zucchini and green pepper and sauté for 7 to 8 minutes with occasional stirring. Add 1 tsp (5 mL) curry powder and cook for 1 minute with constant stirring. Add the bean sprouts and salt, and cook for 2 to 3 minutes. Add the contents of the skillet to the tofu and keep warm in the oven.

3. Add the remaining Garlic-Infused Oil to the skillet over medium heat. Add the remaining curry powder and cook for 1 minute with constant stirring. Pour in the coconut milk, stir and cook over very low heat for 2 to 3 minutes.

4. Put the tofu and vegetables back into the skillet, then mix well with the coconut curry sauce. Heat for a couple of minutes, then season to taste with pepper and serve.

Preparation time:

5 minutes

Cooking time:

5 minutes

Choose a good-quality olive oil. Not only will it taste better, but you will also benefit from its heart-healthy fats.

TIP

The oil keeps for 2 weeks in the refrigerator. When cold, it will solidify. Simply remove it from the fridge 15 minutes before you need it.

Garlic-Infused Oil

2 cups	olive oil, divided	500 mL
1	head garlic, separated into cloves and cloves peeled	1

1. Heat $\frac{1}{4}$ cup (60 mL) oil in a skillet over medium heat. Add the garlic cloves and sauté for 1 minute. Add the remaining oil and reduce heat to medium-low. Cook, stirring, for 2 to 3 minutes to infuse the garlic flavor into the oil.

2. Remove from heat and let the oil cool in the pan. This allows the oil to infuse further. Once the oil has cooled, strain it through a fine-mesh sieve and discard the garlic. Transfer the oil to an airtight container and refrigerate immediately.

Ratatouille with Tofu

MAKES 4 SERVINGS

· MAKE AHEAD ·

Preparation time:

15 minutes

Cooking time:

30 minutes

TIP

This dish may be prepared in advance and stored in an airtight container in the refrigerator for up to 2 days, then reheated. It is not advisable to freeze it, because tofu changes texture when thawed after being frozen.

3½ oz	green beans	100 g
2	zucchini (9 oz/260 g total)	2
1	small eggplant (6½ oz/180 g)	1
1	yellow or red bell pepper	1
1	carrot	1
2 tbsp	Garlic-Infused Oil (page 147)	30 mL
	Salt and freshly ground black pepper	
11½ oz	firm regular tofu, diced	330 g
1¼ cups	canned diced tomatoes, with juice	300 mL
1 tsp	herbes de Provence	5 mL
⅛ tsp	cayenne pepper (optional)	0.5 mL

1. Boil or steam the green beans. Drain, cut them into ¾-inch (2 cm) pieces and set aside.

2. Meanwhile, dice the zucchini, eggplant, yellow pepper and carrot into ⅔-inch (1.5 cm) pieces.

3. Heat the Garlic-Infused Oil in a saucepan over medium heat. Add zucchini, eggplant, yellow pepper and carrot to the saucepan. Season with salt and pepper. Sauté for 8 to 10 minutes, with some stirring.

4. Add the tofu cubes, tomatoes, herbes de Provence and cayenne pepper (if using). Cover and cook over low heat for about 10 minutes, until all vegetables are soft but still a bit al dente. Add the cooked green beans and cook for an additional 2 to 3 minutes. Adjust the seasoning and serve.

NUTRIENTS PER SERVING	
Calories	220
Protein	13 g
Fat	14.0 g
Saturated fat	2.0 g
Carbohydrates	14 g
Fiber	4 g
Sodium	115 mg

Sautéed Tempeh with Mixed Greens

VEGAN

Preparation time:

15 minutes

Standing time:

30 minutes

Cooking time:

15 minutes

TIP

Tempeh can be found in the chilled section of health food stores. Most often it is a compact 8-oz (240 g) square block.

1 lb	tempeh (2 blocks)	480 g
3 tbsp	soy sauce	45 mL
3 tbsp	unseasoned rice vinegar	45 mL
2 tsp	sesame oil	10 mL
2 tbsp	grated gingerroot	30 mL
5 cups	mixed greens (4 oz/120 g)	1.25 L
2 tbsp	Classic Vinaigrette (page 95)	30 mL
	Salt and freshly ground black pepper	
4 tsp	Garlic-Infused Oil (page 147)	20 mL
1	green onion (green part only), chopped	1

1. Slice each tempeh block through the length and cut each piece into 4. Steam the tempeh for 10 minutes.

2. Meanwhile, combine the soy sauce, rice vinegar, sesame oil and ginger in a bowl. Place the warm tempeh in the bowl, then let stand at room temperature for about 30 minutes, turning the tempeh pieces once to cover them well.

3. While tempeh is marinating, wash the greens and spin-dry, then add them to a salad bowl. Pour the Classic Vinaigrette over the greens, season with salt and pepper, then toss well. Distribute the salad onto four serving plates.

4. Heat the Garlic-Infused Oil in a pan over medium-high heat. Add the tempeh pieces and sauté until golden-brown, about 4 minutes. Arrange the tempeh pieces on the salad, garnish with the green onion, then serve.

NUTRIENTS PER SERVING	
Calories	340
Protein	23 g
Fat	23.0 g
Saturated fat	4.0 g
Carbohydrates	15 g
Fiber	12 g
Sodium	150 mg

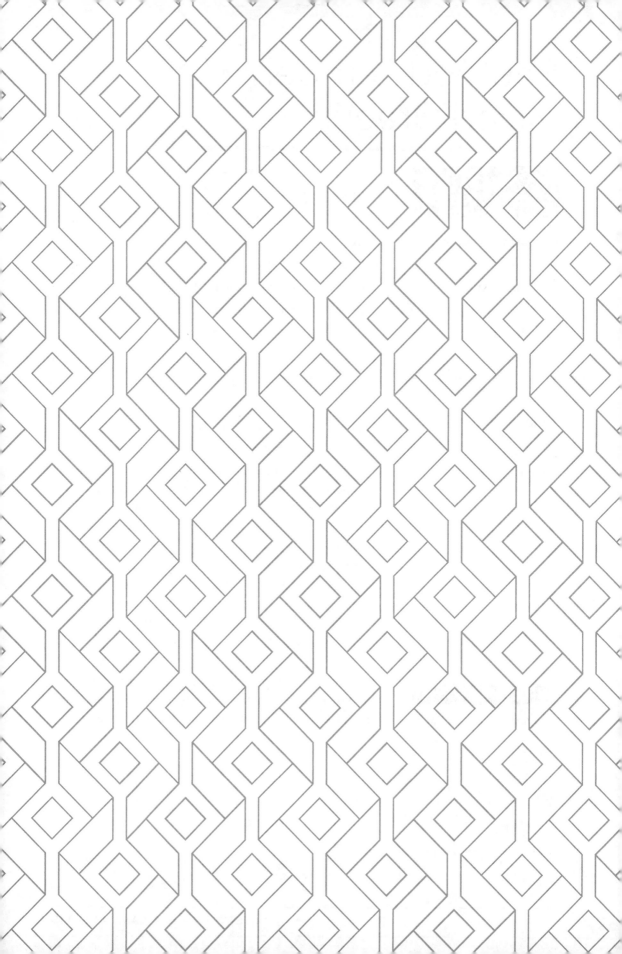

Fish and Seafood

Spaghetti with Citrus and Anchovy Pesto

VEGAN OPTION

Preparation time:

15 minutes

Cooking time:

10 minutes

TIPS

Keep the serving plates in the oven at the lowest setting so they are warm when you serve.

The citrus pesto can be prepared through step 3 and refrigerated for up to 2 days. When ready to serve, proceed with step 4.

• Food processor

10	fresh basil leaves	10
1	orange, peeled	1
1/3 cup	almonds (about 1 1/2 oz/45 g)	75 mL
3 tbsp	drained capers	45 mL
8	anchovy fillets (about 1 oz/30 g total)	8
1 tbsp	freshly squeezed lemon juice	15 mL
1 tbsp	pure maple syrup	15 mL
1/4 cup	extra virgin olive oil	60 mL
	Additional extra virgin olive oil	
11 oz	gluten-free spaghetti	320 g

1. Rinse the basil leaves briefly only if they are very dirty. Otherwise, use a wet towel to clean the leaves, then pat them dry between two paper towels.

2. Drop the peeled orange into the food processor with the almonds, capers, anchovies, basil, lemon juice and maple syrup. Slowly mix in the 1/4 cup (60 mL) olive oil until a creamy but thick consistency is achieved.

3. Transfer the pesto to a small bowl and add olive oil just to cover it, to prevent the oxidation (and darkening) of its surface. Cover the bowl with plastic wrap and chill until ready to use.

4. Cook spaghetti in a large pot of boiling salted water until al dente.

5. While the pasta is cooking, put the citrus pesto in a small bowl, then add around 1/4 cup (60 mL) of pasta cooking water, which will warm up the sauce and dilute it a bit.

6. Drain the spaghetti and add back to the cooking pot. Add the pesto sauce and mix well. Serve in warmed dishes.

Vegan Variation

Simply omit the anchovies.

Provence-Style Cod Casserole

Preparation time:

15 minutes

Cooking time:

55 minutes

A tasty, one-dish dinner. Any other lean, flaky-textured fish may be substituted for cod.

TIP

The cooled casserole may be stored in an airtight container in the refrigerator for up to 3 days. Reheat in the microwave before serving.

NUTRIENTS PER SERVING	
Calories	380
Protein	41 g
Fat	7.0 g
Saturated fat	1.0 g
Carbohydrates	38 g
Fiber	6 g
Sodium	390 mg

- **Preheat oven to 400°F (200°C)**
- **Large baking dish**

4	potatoes (1¾ lbs/800 g total)	4
4	plum (Roma) tomatoes (10 oz/ 280 g total)	4
1¾ lbs	skinless cod or hake fillet, cut into large pieces	800 g
1 tbsp	Garlic-Infused Oil (page 147)	15 mL
12	black olives	12
1 tbsp	dried oregano	15 mL
	Salt and freshly ground black pepper	
1⅓ cups	Allergen-Free Vegetable Broth (page 116)	325 mL

1. Peel the potatoes, then cut them into ¼-inch (0.5 cm) thick slices. Cut the tomatoes into ¼-inch (0.5 cm) thick slices.

2. Cover the bottom of a baking dish with about half of the potato slices. Add the tomatoes. Lay the cod pieces over the tomatoes, then drizzle with the Garlic-Infused Oil. Add the olives and the oregano. Season with salt and pepper. Pour in the broth and cover with the remaining potato slices.

3. Cover and bake in the middle of the preheated oven until the potatoes are fully cooked, about 50 to 55 minutes. For a nice golden crust, uncover and turn on the broiler for the last 2 minutes. Serve directly out of the baking dish.

Blackened Fish Fillets

• MAKE AHEAD •

Preparation time:

10 minutes

Cooking time:

10 minutes

This is a classic Louisiana method of cooking with a spicy coating, which can be used for poultry, meat or fish. At the end of cooking, the coating should begin to blacken slightly at the edges.

TIP

The cooked fish fillets may be stored in an airtight container in the refrigerator for up to 3 days. Reheat in the microwave before serving.

NUTRIENTS PER SERVING	
Calories	240
Protein	38 g
Fat	7.0 g
Saturated fat	1.5 g
Carbohydrates	9 g
Fiber	3 g
Sodium	350 mg

• **Preheat greased barbecue grill to high (optional)**

2 tbsp	paprika	30 mL
1 tsp	dried oregano	5 mL
1 tsp	cayenne pepper	5 mL
1 tsp	granulated sugar	5 mL
½ tsp	salt	2 mL
¾ tsp	freshly ground black pepper	3 mL
2 tbsp	cornmeal (optional)	30 mL
4	skinless tilapia or turbot fillets (about 1½ lbs/700 g total)	4
3 tbsp	canola oil (optional)	45 mL
2	cloves garlic (optional)	2
1	lemon, cut into wedges	1

1. In a shallow bowl, stir together the paprika, oregano, cayenne pepper, sugar, salt and pepper. To obtain a crispier crust, add the cornmeal.

2. Pat the fillets dry and dredge them in the mixture, turning them to coat well. Shake off and discard the excess.

3. Place the fillets on the preheated grill. Cook until the fish is opaque throughout and lightly blackened on the outside, 4 to 5 minutes per side, turning once. (Alternatively, heat the oil in a large skillet over medium-high heat. Add the garlic and sauté until it is golden-brown, about 2 minutes. Discard the garlic, add the fish, then fry for 4 to 5 minutes on each side or until it is cooked through and lightly blackened on the outside.)

4. Serve immediately with the lemon wedges.

Vegetable Salad with Mackerel

Preparation time:

15 minutes

Cooking time:

15 minutes

Inexpensive and easy to prepare, mackerel is a good source of omega-3s.

TIP

The salad, without the tomatoes, can be covered and refrigerated for up to 2 days. Add the tomatoes just before serving.

3	potatoes (1¼ lbs/600 g total)	3
5 oz	green beans	140 g
2	tomatoes, diced	2
8½ oz	canned mackerel	240 g
⅓ cup	Classic Vinaigrette (page 95)	75 mL
	Salt and freshly ground black pepper	

1. Peel the potatoes and cut them in half. Place them in a steamer basket or in a pot of salted water to either steam or boil for 13 minutes.

2. Meanwhile, trim the ends of the green beans. Add the green beans to the potatoes and continue steaming or boiling for another 7 minutes, until the potatoes are tender and the beans are tender-crisp. Let the vegetables cool down for 10 minutes or longer, so they won't be so hot to handle.

3. Cut the potatoes and green beans into bite-size pieces and put them in a salad bowl. Add tomatoes to the bowl. Drain the mackerel fillets and add them to the bowl. Pour the Classic Vinaigrette over the salad, then season with salt and pepper to taste. Toss the salad and serve.

NUTRIENTS PER SERVING	
Calories	360
Protein	17 g
Fat	20.0 g
Saturated fat	3.5 g
Carbohydrates	30 g
Fiber	3 g
Sodium	260 mg

Salmon with a Spicy Crust

• MAKE AHEAD •

Preparation time:

10 minutes

Cooking time:

10 minutes

TIPS

Keep the serving plates warm on the stove while you're preparing the dish.

The cooked fish fillets may be stored in an airtight container in the refrigerator for up to 3 days. Reheat in the microwave before serving.

NUTRIENTS PER SERVING		
Calories		320
Protein		32 g
Fat		19.0 g
Saturated fat		2.0 g
Carbohydrates		6 g
Fiber		2 g
Sodium		370 mg

- **Preheat oven to 450°F (230°C)**
- **Pepper mill or spice grinder (optional)**

2 tsp	whole black peppercorns	10 mL
2 tbsp	whole coriander seeds	30 mL
2 tbsp	mustard seeds	30 mL
2 tbsp	celery seeds	30 mL
³⁄₄ tsp	salt	3 mL
1¼ lbs	skinless salmon fillet, cut into 4 pieces	600 g
¼ cup	canola oil	60 mL

1. Coarsely grind the peppercorns, coriander, mustard and celery seeds using a pepper mill or spice grinder if available. Otherwise, place the spices in a plastic bag and crush them using a rolling pin. Transfer the mixture to a shallow dish, add the salt, then coat the salmon pieces on both sides with the spice mixture.

2. Heat the oil in a nonstick skillet over medium heat. Add the salmon and cook until the crust is golden, about 1 to 2 minutes per side, taking care not to let it burn.

3. Transfer the fillets to a baking dish, place the dish in the middle of the preheated oven and bake for about 7 to 8 minutes for a ³⁄₄- to 1-inch (2 to 2.5 cm) thick fillet. Since the cooking time depends on the thickness of the fillets and the actual temperature of the oven, it is important to check with a fork to see if the fish is cooked through; the fish is done when it flakes easily and does not stick to the prongs. Serve on warmed plates.

Baked Salmon with Herbs

Preparation time:

5 minutes

Cooking time:

10 minutes

This recipe is quick, easy, tasty and full of omega-3s, an essential fatty acid.

TIP

The cooked fish fillets may be stored in an airtight container in the refrigerator for up to 3 days or in the freezer for up to 1 month. Thaw in the refrigerator, if necessary, then reheat in the microwave before serving.

NUTRIENTS PER SERVING	
Calories	220
Protein	30 g
Fat	10.2 g
Saturated fat	2.2 g
Carbohydrates	1 g
Fiber	0 g
Sodium	75 mg

- Preheat oven to 425°F (220°C)
- Rimmed baking sheet, oiled

1¼ lbs	salmon fillet	600 g
2 tbsp	olive oil	30 mL
	Salt and freshly ground black pepper	
2 tbsp	dried oregano	30 mL

1. Cut the salmon fillet into 4 equal pieces. Put them on the prepared baking sheet and brush them with oil. Add salt and pepper, then cover with oregano.

2. Place in the middle of the preheated oven and bake for about 10 minutes for a ¾- to 1-inch (2 to 2.5 cm) thick fillet. Since the cooking time depends on the fillet thickness and the actual temperature of the oven, it is important to check with a fork to see if the fish is cooked through; the fish is done when it flakes easily and does not stick to the prongs. Serve on warmed plates.

Curried Trout

Preparation time:

5 minutes

Cooking time:

10 minutes

A very simple recipe. For good results, use only the freshest fish and a high-quality curry powder.

TIPS

Keep the serving plates in the oven at the lowest setting so they are warm when you serve.

Like all spices, curry can be stored in an airtight container in a cool, dry place for 6 months maximum.

4	trout fillets (about 1½ lbs/700 g total)	4
1 tbsp	curry powder	15 mL
2 tbsp	olive oil	30 mL
	Salt and freshly ground black pepper	

1. Evenly coat the fillets with the curry powder (slightly less on the skin side).

2. Heat the oil in a frying pan. When the pan is hot, add the fillets, skin side down. Cook for 4 to 5 minutes, then lower the heat, turn the fillets and continue to cook for 3 to 4 minutes, until the flesh is tender and opaque. Check with a fork to see if it is cooked through; the fish is done when it flakes easily and does not stick to the prongs.

3. Peel and discard the skin from the top of the fillets. Add salt and pepper to taste, then serve on warmed plates.

NUTRIENTS PER SERVING

Calories	320
Protein	38 g
Fat	17.0 g
Saturated fat	3.0 g
Carbohydrates	1 g
Fiber	1 g
Sodium	95 mg

Asian Shrimp Soup

**MAKES
4 SERVINGS**

Preparation time:

10 minutes

Cooking time:

10 minutes

5½ oz	rice stick noodles	160 g
28	medium-large shrimp (about 10 oz/ 280 g total), peeled and deveined	28
2	carrots, grated	2
1¼ cups	thinly sliced savoy cabbage	300 mL
6 cups	Allergen-Free Vegetable Broth (page 116)	1.5 L
2 tsp	grated gingerroot	10 mL
1	dried chile pepper, minced	1
	Salt	
¼ cup	freshly squeezed lime juice	60 mL
4 tsp	fresh cilantro leaves	20 mL

1. Cook the rice stick noodles in a pot of salted boiling water for 4 minutes or according to package directions. Drain and set aside.

2. Meanwhile, in a saucepan of salted boiling water, boil the shrimp for about 3 minutes, until they become pink. Drain and set aside.

3. Portion out carrots and cabbage into 4 individual serving bowls with a capacity of at least 2 cups (500 mL). Add the cooked rice stick noodles to the bowls.

4. Heat the broth in a saucepan. Add the grated ginger and chile pepper. Cook for 2 minutes. Add the cooked shrimp and cook for an additional 3 to 4 minutes. Adjust the seasoning if needed.

5. Pour the hot broth into the serving bowls. Add the lime juice, garnish with whole cilantro leaves and serve.

NUTRIENTS PER SERVING

Calories	330
Protein	17 g
Fat	7.0 g
Saturated fat	1.0 g
Carbohydrates	51 g
Fiber	6 g
Sodium	780 mg

Vegan Variation

Tofu may be substituted for the shrimp. To give the tofu more flavor, marinate it in a few tbsp (30 to 45 mL) of soy sauce and sesame oil for a few minutes, then sauté it in a hot pan before adding it to the soup.

Shrimp and Arugula Quinoa Salad

VEGAN OPTION

· MAKE AHEAD ·

Preparation time:

15 minutes

Cooking time:

15 minutes

Standing time:

20 minutes

1 cup	quinoa	250 mL
2 cups	water	500 mL
	Salt	
$\frac{1}{2}$	bunch arugula ($2\frac{3}{4}$ oz/80 g), coarsely chopped	$\frac{1}{2}$
2 cups	mini tomatoes (10 oz/280 g), halved	500 mL
2 tbsp	drained capers	30 mL
$\frac{1}{4}$ cup	extra virgin olive oil	60 mL
4 tsp	freshly squeezed lemon juice	20 mL
1 tsp	grated gingerroot	5 mL
Pinch	cayenne pepper	Pinch
	Freshly ground black pepper	
40	small shrimp (about $7\frac{1}{2}$ oz/ 220 g total), cooked	40
$\frac{1}{4}$ cup	finely chopped fresh chives	60 mL

1. Place the quinoa in a fine-mesh strainer and hold it under cold running water until the water runs clear, then drain well.

2. Combine the quinoa, water and a pinch of salt in a saucepan. Bring to a boil, then reduce to a simmer. Cover and cook until the grains are translucent and the germ has spiraled out from each grain, about 15 minutes. Let it cool down for 10 minutes.

3. Put the arugula, tomatoes and capers in a salad bowl. Add the cooked quinoa.

NUTRIENTS PER SERVING

Calories	330
Protein	17 g
Fat	17.0 g
Saturated fat	2.5 g
Carbohydrates	28 g
Fiber	4 g
Sodium	270 mg

4. Put the oil, lemon juice, grated ginger, cayenne pepper, and salt and pepper to taste in a small bowl. Whisk, using a fork, until combined. Pour over the salad.

5. Gently toss to combine. Add the shrimp and sprinkle with the finely chopped chives. Cover and chill for at least 20 minutes before serving to allow the flavors to meld.

Vegan Variation

Swap the shrimp for tempeh. Use your favorite tempeh recipe or use ours on page 149.

Singapore Noodles

**MAKES
4 SERVINGS**

• **MAKE AHEAD** •

Preparation time:

15 minutes

Cooking time:

20 minutes

*Curried noodles are
a classic in Southeast
Asia, particularly
in Singapore, where
Chinese cuisine is
influenced by Indian
culture. This recipe
is one of numerous
versions, all made with
either rice or wheat
noodles, various types
of meat and seasonings,
but always spiced up
with curry.*

10 oz	rice stick noodles	280 g
2 tbsp	soy sauce	30 mL
2 tbsp	fish sauce (nam pla)	30 mL
3 tbsp	Garlic-Infused Oil (page 147), divided	45 mL
7 oz	boneless pork loin, cut into strips	200 g
24	small shrimp (about 4½ oz/130 g total), peeled and deveined	24
1	green bell pepper, finely chopped	1
½	dried chile pepper, minced	½
1 tbsp	grated gingerroot	15 mL
1 tbsp	curry powder	15 mL
1 tbsp	granulated sugar	15 mL
¼ cup	peanuts (optional)	60 mL
2 tbsp	chopped fresh cilantro (optional)	30 mL

1. Cook the rice stick noodles in a large pot of salted boiling water until they are al dente, about 3 minutes or according to package directions. Rinse the noodles in cold water to stop the cooking process and drain thoroughly. Set aside.

2. Mix the soy sauce and fish sauce in a small bowl. Set aside.

3. Heat 1 tbsp (15 mL) of the Garlic-Infused Oil in a wok or skillet over high heat. Add the pork and cook, stirring constantly, until it is lightly browned, about 4 minutes. Remove the pork from the pan using a slotted spoon and set aside on a plate.

4. Add the shrimp to the wok or skillet and cook, with some stirring, until the shrimp lose their gray color and turn pink, 3 to 4 minutes. Set the shrimp aside on the plate with the pork.

NUTRIENTS PER SERVING

Calories	470
Protein	20 g
Fat	13.0 g
Saturated fat	2.5 g
Carbohydrates	65 g
Fiber	3 g
Sodium	990 mg

This dish can be prepared through step 6, then stored in an airtight container in the refrigerator for up to 3 days. Reheat in the microwave before continuing with step 7.

Keep the serving plates in the oven at the lowest setting so they are warm when you serve.

5. Add the remaining Garlic-Infused Oil to the wok or skillet. Add the green pepper and cook, stirring occasionally, for about 5 minutes. Stir in the ginger and chile pepper. Cook for 1 minute, stirring. Add the curry powder and sugar. Cook for a few seconds, stirring, then pour in the noodles. Cook for 1 minute with some stirring. Add the soy mixture.

6. Return the pork and shrimp to the skillet. Pour in about $1/3$ cup (75 mL) water to allow the noodles to separate. Continue cooking, with occasional stirring, until the noodles start to turn golden-colored, 5 to 7 minutes.

7. Adjust the seasoning, garnish with the peanuts and cilantro (if using), then serve on warmed dishes.

Vegan Variation

Omit the fish sauce and swap the pork and shrimp for tempeh. Use your favorite tempeh recipe or use ours on page 149.

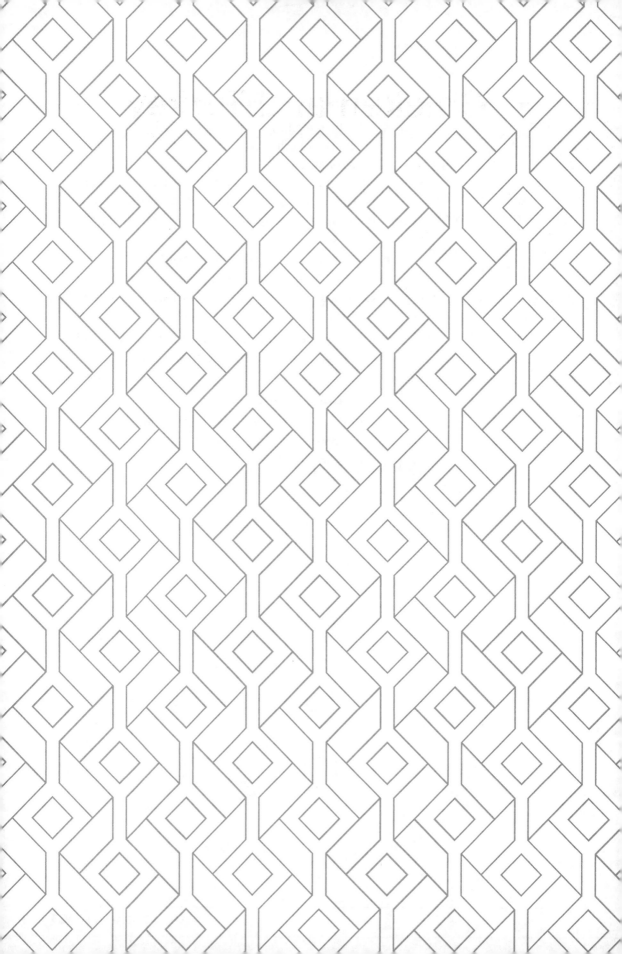

Chicken and Turkey

Chicken Salad with a Coriander-Mustard Dressing

VEGAN OPTION

Preparation time:

10 minutes

Marinating time:

8 hours

Cooking time:

20 minutes

½ cup	olive oil	125 mL
¼ cup	freshly squeezed lemon juice	60 mL
1 tbsp	whole-grain mustard	15 mL
1 tbsp	sesame oil	15 mL
¾ tsp	coriander seeds, crushed	3 mL
2	boneless skinless chicken breasts (about 1¼ lbs/600 g total)	2
5½ oz	green beans	160 g
2	carrots	2
½	head Boston lettuce	½
4	slices bacon (about 2¾ oz/80 g total), chopped	4
	Salt and freshly ground black pepper	
2 tbsp	fresh cilantro leaves (optional)	30 mL

1. In a small bowl, combine the olive oil, lemon juice, mustard, sesame oil and coriander seeds.

2. Put the chicken breasts in a shallow dish. Pour about half of the dressing over the chicken (just enough to cover). Cover and marinate overnight in the refrigerator. Refrigerate the remaining marinade to be used as a salad dressing.

3. Preheat barbecue grill to medium or preheat broiler.

4. Boil the green beans for 7 to 8 minutes in a pot of salted boiling water, then immerse in cold water to stop the cooking and fix the color.

5. Julienne the carrots into matchstick-sized pieces. Tear the lettuce into small pieces and arrange onto four individual serving plates. Mix the green beans and carrots in a bowl.

NUTRIENTS PER SERVING

Calories	320
Protein	38 g
Fat	14.0 g
Saturated fat	2.5 g
Carbohydrates	10 g
Fiber	3 g
Sodium	270 mg

Chicken breasts and bacon can be cooked 1 to 2 days in advance. Assemble the salad right before serving.

6. In a nonstick skillet, fry the chopped bacon until crisp. Transfer the bacon to a paper towel to absorb the excess fat, then add it to the bowl with the vegetables.

7. Cook the chicken breasts on preheated grill (or place them on a broiler pan and broil) for 10 to 12 minutes, basting occasionally with some of the marinade and turning them once, until no longer pink inside. Transfer to a cutting board. Season with salt and pepper. Slice the breasts on a bias into thin pieces.

8. Pour the reserved unused dressing over the green beans and carrots and season with salt and pepper to taste, mixing well. Distribute the vegetables over the lettuce on the serving plates.

9. Arrange the chicken pieces on top of each plate. Garnish with fresh cilantro leaves.

Vegan Variation

Omit the bacon and swap the chicken for tempeh. Tempeh can be marinated for a couple of hours instead of overnight.

Grilled Chicken Caesar Salad

MAKES 4 SERVINGS

• MAKE AHEAD •

Preparation time:

20 minutes

Cooking time:

15 minutes

•	**Preheat barbecue grill to medium-high heat or preheat broiler**	
2	small bone-in skinless chicken breasts (about 1¾ lbs/800 g total)	2
⅓ cup	Garlic-Infused Oil (page 147), divided	75 mL
4	anchovy fillets	4
2	large egg yolks (see tip)	2
¼ tsp	hot pepper sauce, such as Tabasco	1 mL
2 tbsp	wine vinegar	30 mL
2 tsp	Dijon mustard	10 mL
2	slices bacon (about 1½ oz/40 g total), chopped	2
1	head romaine lettuce (1 lb, 3 oz/ 550 g), torn into bite-size pieces	1
	Salt and freshly ground black pepper	

1. Pat the chicken dry, then brush it with 2 tsp (10 mL) of the Garlic-Infused Oil and season with salt and pepper. Grill or broil the chicken until cooked through and golden-colored, about 15 minutes, turning it once. Transfer the chicken to a cutting board and cover it loosely with foil.

2. Drain the anchovy fillets, pat them dry on a paper towel, then mince.

3. In a small saucepan, heat 1 tbsp (15 mL) Garlic-Infused Oil over medium-low heat. Add the minced anchovies, then stir and mash them for 1 minute to help them melt. Set aside.

NUTRIENTS PER SERVING

Calories	370
Protein	41 g
Fat	21.0 g
Saturated fat	4.0 g
Carbohydrates	4 g
Fiber	3 g
Sodium	330 mg

TIP

The egg yolks in this recipe are used raw. If the food safety of raw eggs is a concern for you, use pasteurized-in-shell egg yolks.

4. In a bowl, whisk together the egg yolks, hot pepper sauce, vinegar and mustard. Add the remaining Garlic-Infused Oil in a stream, whisking until the dressing is emulsified. Add the anchovy-garlic oil. Add salt and pepper to taste. Set aside.

5. In a nonstick skillet, fry the chopped bacon until crisp. Set aside on a paper towel to absorb the excess fat.

6. In a salad bowl, toss the romaine lettuce with the bacon bits and the dressing until the salad is well combined. Cut the chicken crosswise into thin slices, then arrange the slices over the salad and serve.

Vegan Variation

Omit the anchovies, egg yolks and bacon and swap the chicken for tempeh. Use your favorite tempeh recipe or use ours on page 149.

Grilled Chicken in Coconut Milk with Spices

VEGAN OPTION

Preparation time:

15 minutes

Marinating time:

30 minutes

Cooking time:

15 minutes

This Indian recipe is beautifully scented and not piquant, which makes it a great hit with everybody.

• Blender or food processor

2 tbsp	grated gingerroot	30 mL
1⅓ cups	light coconut milk	325 mL
1 tsp	ground cumin	5 mL
¾ tsp	ground turmeric	3 mL
2	whole cloves	2
½ tsp	anise seeds	2 mL
⅛ tsp	whole black peppercorns	0.5 mL
1	cardamom pod	1
Pinch	freshly grated nutmeg	Pinch
1	large boneless skinless chicken breast (about 14 oz/400 g)	1
	Salt	
1½ tbsp	chopped fresh cilantro (optional)	22 mL

1. In blender or food processor, combine the ginger, coconut milk, cumin, turmeric, cloves, anise seeds and black peppercorns. Split the cardamom pod open to extract the seeds: remove and discard the pod, then add the seeds to the blender. Add a pinch of freshly grated nutmeg. Blend to a smooth paste.

2. Cut chicken breast on the diagonal into 4 thick slices. Arrange it in a shallow dish. Add half of the coconut milk mixture and toss well to coat the chicken evenly. Cover the dish and marinate for at least 30 minutes at room temperature, or overnight in the refrigerator. Keep the remaining sauce separate in the refrigerator.

NUTRIENTS PER SERVING	
Calories	190
Protein	23 g
Fat	9.0 g
Saturated fat	7.0 g
Carbohydrates	4 g
Fiber	0 g
Sodium	60 mg

Most spices, excluding onion and garlic powder, are low in FODMAPs. Don't hesitate to use them to add flavor to your dishes.

3. Preheat barbecue grill to medium-high heat or preheat broiler.

4. Remove chicken from marinade, discarding excess marinade. Cook the chicken on a medium grill for 12 to 15 minutes, turning once, until browned and no longer pink inside. (Alternatively, place chicken on broiler pan and broil.)

5. Meanwhile, pour the remaining coconut mixture into a saucepan and bring to a boil, stirring occasionally. Adjust the seasoning, adding salt only if necessary.

6. Serve the chicken on individual plates with the sauce. Garnish with chopped cilantro (if using).

Vegan Variation

Swap the chicken for cubed tofu.

Chicken Souvlaki

Preparation time:

20 minutes

Standing time:

3 hours

Cooking time:

15 minutes

*Souvlaki is a Greek
specialty consisting of
meat chunks that have
been marinated in a
mixture of oil, lemon
juice, oregano and
seasonings, then grilled
and served with tzatziki.*

NUTRIENTS PER SERVING	
Calories	450
Protein	42 g
Fat	17.0 g
Saturated fat	4.5 g
Carbohydrates	32 g
Fiber	3 g
Sodium	330 mg

- 2 fine-mesh sieves
- 4 or 8 skewers, soaked if necessary

2 tbsp	freshly squeezed lemon juice	30 mL
4 tbsp	Garlic-Infused Oil (page 147), divided	60 mL
	Salt	
$\frac{3}{4}$ tsp	freshly ground black pepper	3 mL
2 tsp	dried oregano	10 mL
$1\frac{1}{4}$ lbs	boneless skinless chicken breasts, cut into bite-size pieces	600 g
1	medium cucumber	1
2 cups	lactose-free plain yogurt	500 mL
2 tbsp	white wine vinegar	30 mL
$\frac{1}{4}$ cup	chopped fresh mint	60 mL
4	6-inch (15 cm) corn tortillas	4

1. In a shallow dish, mix the lemon juice, 2 tbsp (30 mL) Garlic-Infused Oil, $\frac{1}{2}$ tsp (2 mL) salt, pepper and oregano. Add chicken pieces to the dish, turning to coat them well. Cover and refrigerate for at least 3 hours, turning the pieces once.

2. Meanwhile, peel the cucumber, cut it in half and scrape out seeds. Reserve half the skin; set aside. Grate the cucumber coarsely and place the pieces in a sieve, add a pinch of salt, and let drain for about 30 minutes. Squeeze the pulp to extract liquid and wrap in paper towels to dry.

3. Meanwhile, pour the yogurt into another fine-mesh sieve. Let drain for 30 minutes.

4. Place the cucumber pulp in a bowl, add the drained yogurt, vinegar, remaining Garlic-Infused Oil and a pinch of salt. Whisk well. Chop the reserved cucumber skin, then add to the bowl with mint and mix. Chill, covered, until ready to serve, at least 1 hour.

5. Preheat barbecue grill to medium or preheat broiler.

6. Remove chicken from marinade; discard marinade. Thread the chicken pieces onto skewers and grill until the meat is lightly charred on the surface and chicken is no longer pink inside, about 10 minutes, turning the skewers as needed. (Alternatively, put the chicken pieces on the rack of a broiler pan and broil 3 to 4 inches/8 to 10 cm from the heat for about 10 minutes, turning them over a few times, until no longer pink inside.)

7. Serve the chicken souvlaki with the tzatziki and tortillas.

Japanese-Style Chicken Skewers

MAKES 4 SERVINGS

· MAKE AHEAD ·

· FREEZABLE ·

Preparation time:

15 minutes

Marinating time:

1 hour

Cooking time:

10 minutes

"Yakitori" is the name of these chicken skewers in Japan. I have adapted the original marinade recipe by replacing the sake and mirin (both alcoholic beverages made from rice) with white wine.

NUTRIENTS PER SERVING	
Calories	170
Protein	22 g
Fat	8.0 g
Saturated fat	0.3 g
Carbohydrates	3 g
Fiber	1 g
Sodium	125 mg

- **4 or 8 skewers, soaked if necessary**

1	dried chile pepper, minced	1
1¼ tsp	coriander seeds, coarsely ground	6 mL
1¼ tsp	ground cumin	6 mL
	Freshly ground black pepper	
3 tbsp	soy sauce	45 mL
¼ cup	white wine	60 mL
1 tsp	sesame oil	5 mL
5 tsp	packed brown sugar	25 mL
3 tbsp	freshly squeezed lemon juice	45 mL
8	boneless skinless chicken thighs (about 1 lb, 2 oz/500 g total)	8
1 tbsp	sesame seeds	15 mL

1. Combine the chile pepper, coriander seeds, cumin, pepper to taste, soy sauce, wine, sesame oil, brown sugar and lemon juice in a bowl.

2. Cut the chicken into ¾- to 1-inch (2 to 2.5 cm) pieces and put them in the marinade; mix well. Cover and let stand in the refrigerator for at least 1 hour.

3. Meanwhile, preheat barbecue grill to medium or preheat broiler.

TIP

Chile peppers do not contain any FODMAPs. For some people, they can, however, cause symptoms. Test your tolerance and adjust the quantities as needed.

4. Thread the chicken pieces onto skewers and grill for about 6 to 8 minutes, until the pieces are nicely colored and chicken is no longer pink inside, turning the skewers a couple of times. (Alternatively, put the skewers on a baking sheet and broil $2\frac{1}{2}$ to 4 inches/ 7 to 10 cm from the heat for about 6 to 8 minutes, turning the skewers a few times.)

5. Meanwhile, put the sesame seeds in a small pan and heat over medium heat for a few minutes, stirring until lightly colored.

6. When the chicken is ready, sprinkle with the toasted sesame seeds, then serve.

Vegan Variation

Replace the chicken with firm regular tofu. Remove as much water as possible from the tofu before using, to ensure that it takes in plenty of flavor.

Chicken Piccata

Preparation time:

10 minutes

Cooking time:

15 minutes

Hailing from Italy, piccata consists of seasoned and floured veal or chicken scallops that are quickly sautéed then served with a lemon juice and parsley sauce.

- Preheat oven to 170°F (77°C)
- Meat mallet or rolling pin

2	boneless skinless chicken breasts (about 1¼ lbs/600 g total)	2
	Salt and freshly ground black pepper	
¼ cup	cornstarch	60 mL
1 tbsp	canola oil	15 mL
¼ cup	non-hydrogenated margarine, divided	60 mL
¼ cup	freshly squeezed lemon juice	60 mL
⅓ cup	Allergen-Free Vegetable Broth (page 116)	75 mL
2 tbsp	drained capers	30 mL
1 tbsp	chopped fresh Italian (flat-leaf) parsley	15 mL

1. Cut the chicken breasts in half lengthwise and butterfly them to make cutlets. Flatten and tenderize the cutlets using a meat mallet. Season the cutlets with salt and pepper, then coat them with the cornstarch and shake off the excess.

2. Heat the oil and half of the margarine in a large skillet over medium-high heat, taking care not to let the margarine burn. When the margarine and oil start to sizzle, add a few chicken cutlets at a time and cook for 3 minutes. When the chicken has browned, flip and cook the other side for 3 minutes. Remove and transfer the cutlets to a plate. Cover with foil and put them in the oven to keep them warm. Repeat with the remaining chicken cutlets.

3. Reduce the heat to medium-low and pour in the lemon juice, broth and capers. Bring the mixture to a boil, scraping up brown bits from the pan for extra flavor. Adjust the seasoning. Return all of the chicken to the skillet, cover and simmer for 3 to 4 minutes. Remove the chicken and transfer it to a serving platter.

4. Add the remaining margarine to the skillet and whisk vigorously. Pour the sauce over the chicken and garnish with the chopped parsley. Serve.

NUTRIENTS PER SERVING	
Calories	300
Protein	34 g
Fat	13.0 g
Saturated fat	2.0 g
Carbohydrates	10 g
Fiber	1 g
Sodium	250 mg

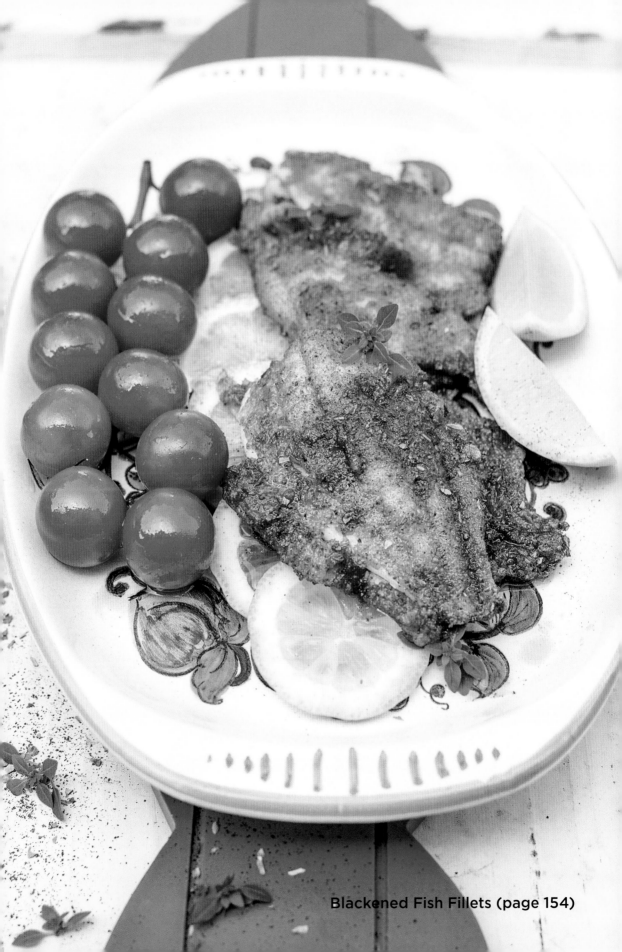

Blackened Fish Fillets (page 154)

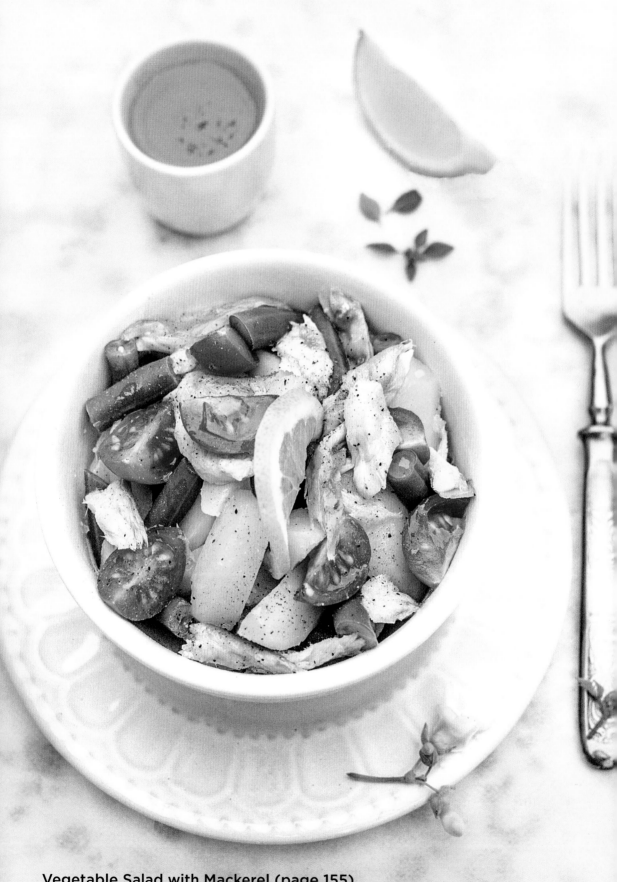

Vegetable Salad with Mackerel (page 155)

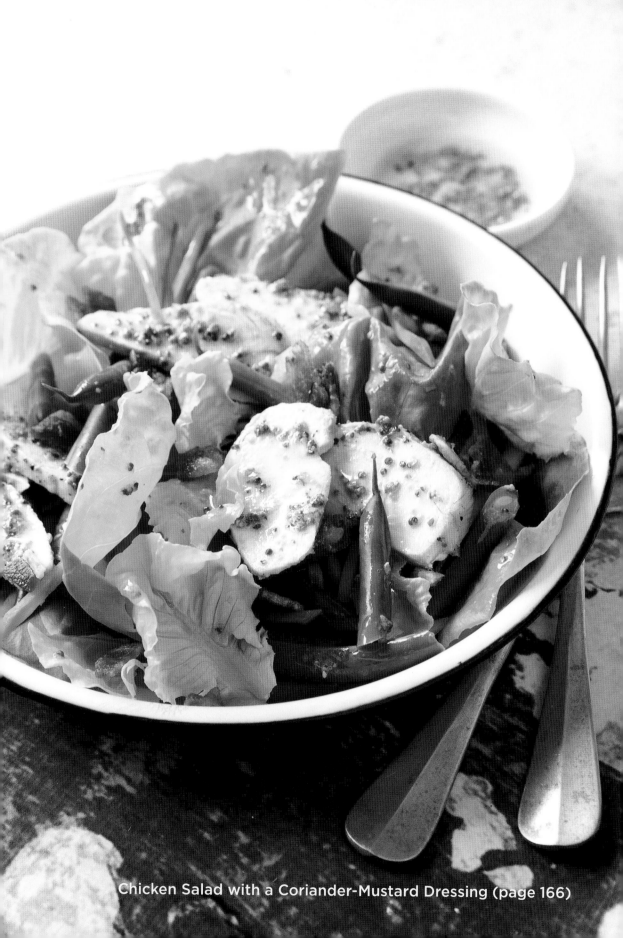

Chicken Salad with a Coriander-Mustard Dressing (page 166)

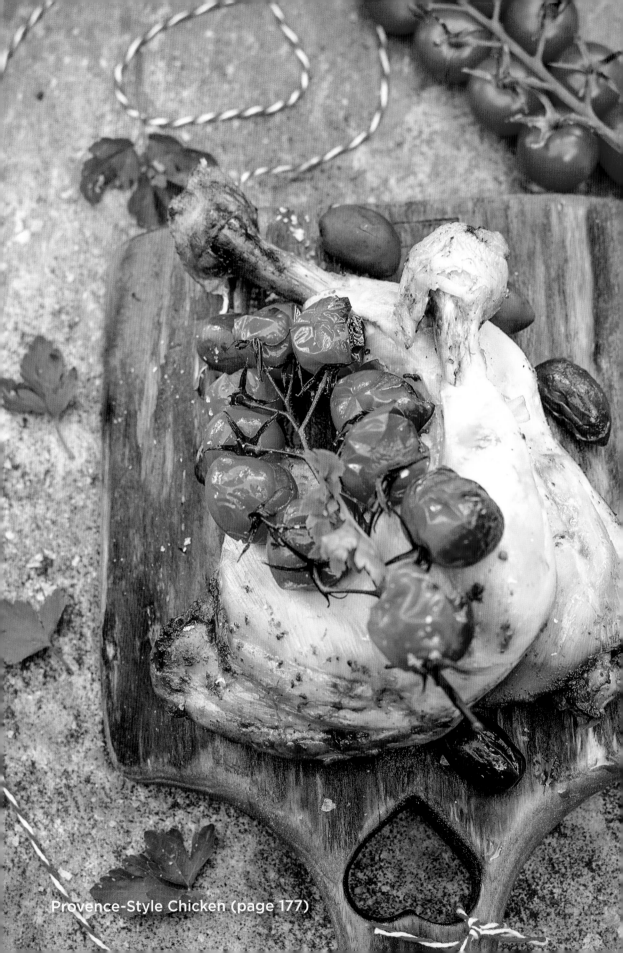
Provence-Style Chicken (page 177)

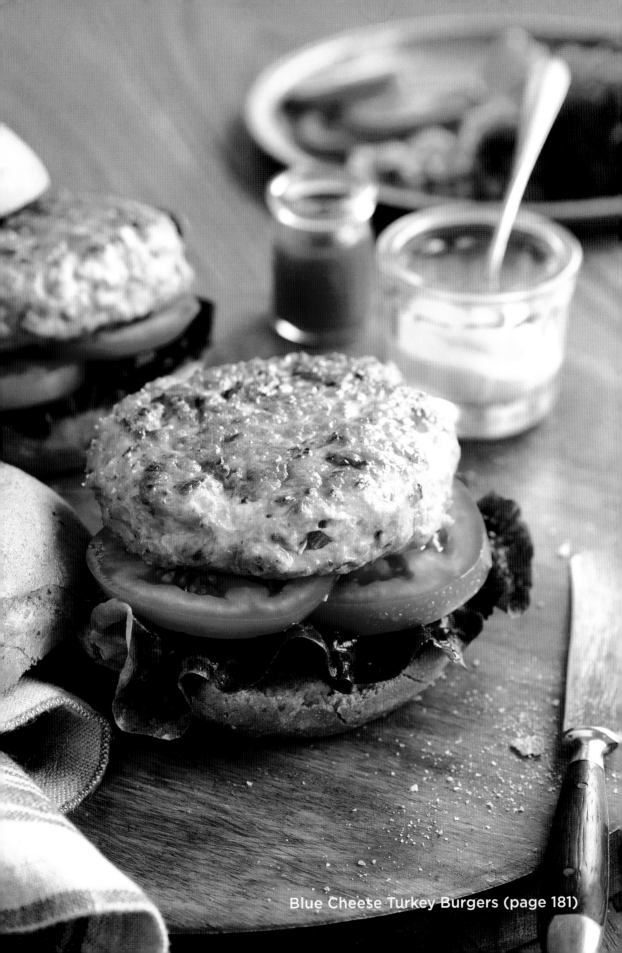

Blue Cheese Turkey Burgers (page 181)

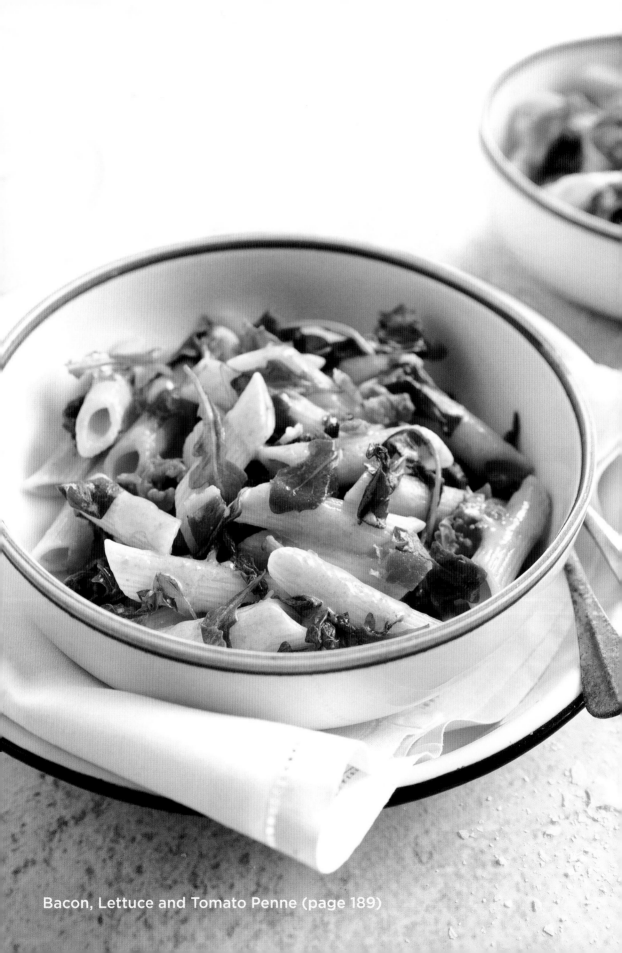

Bacon, Lettuce and Tomato Penne (page 189)

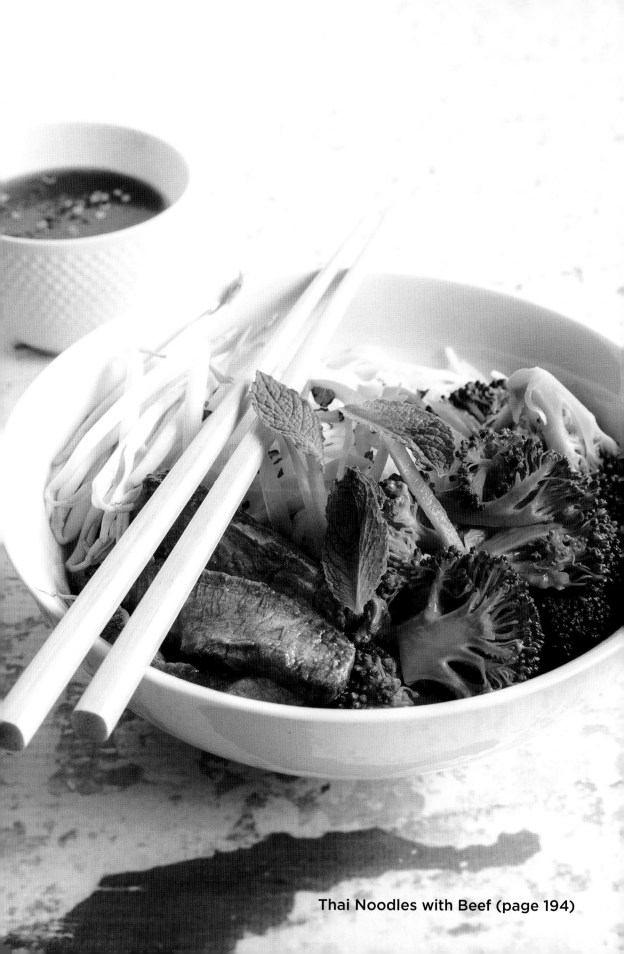

Thai Noodles with Beef (page 194)

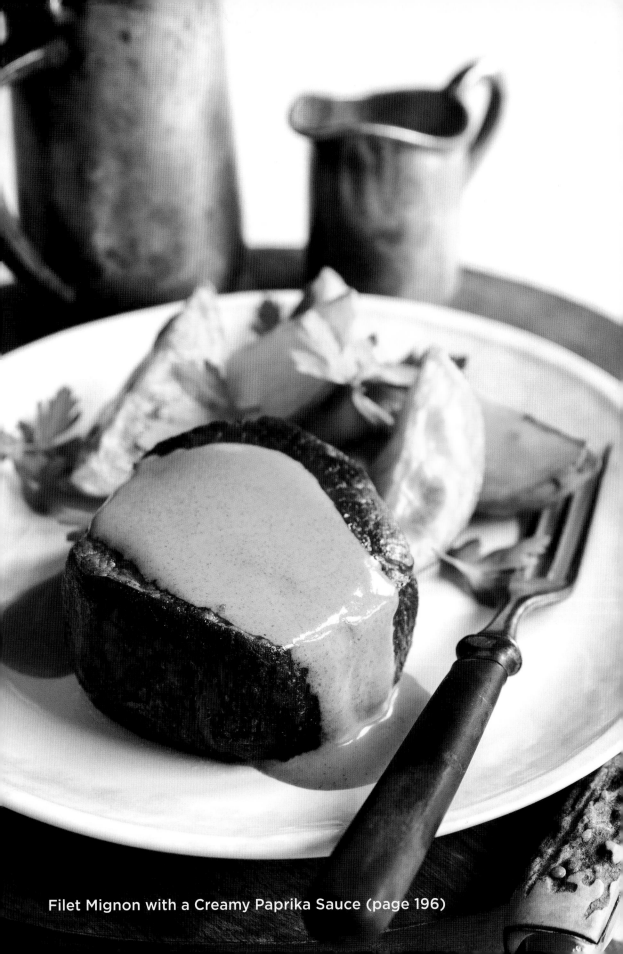

Filet Mignon with a Creamy Paprika Sauce (page 196)

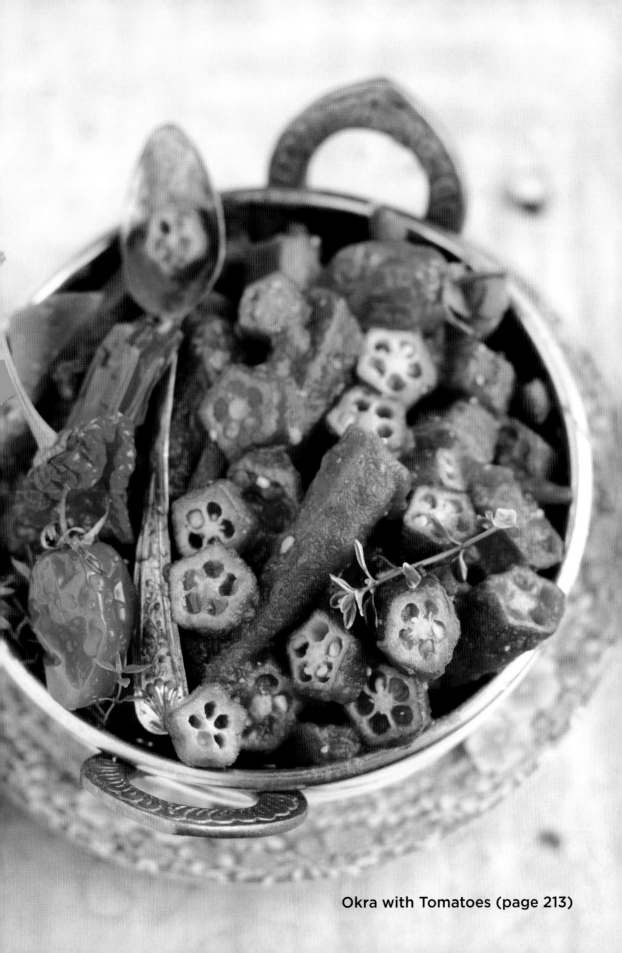

Okra with Tomatoes (page 213)

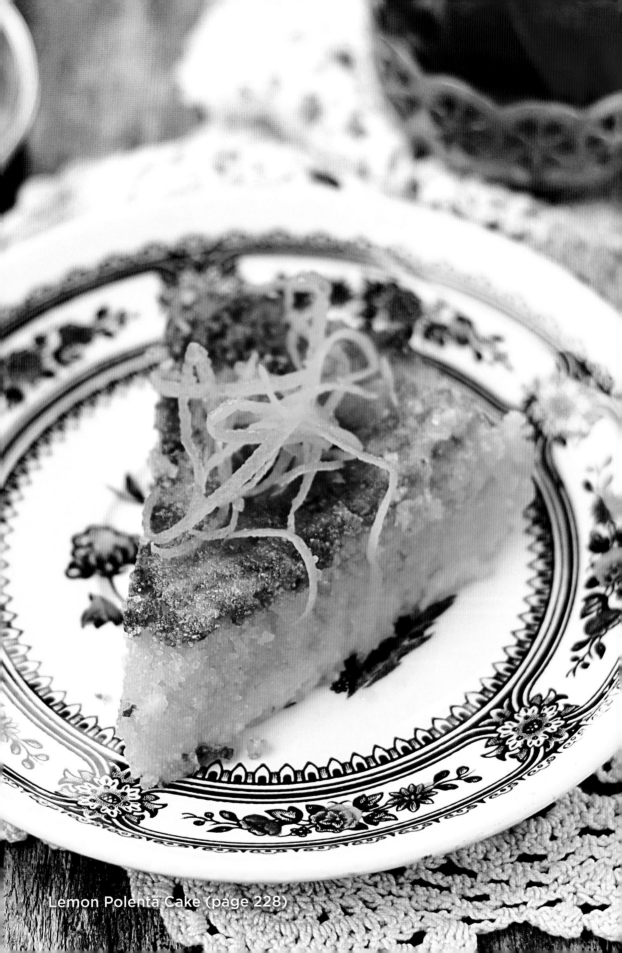

Lemon Polenta Cake (page 228)

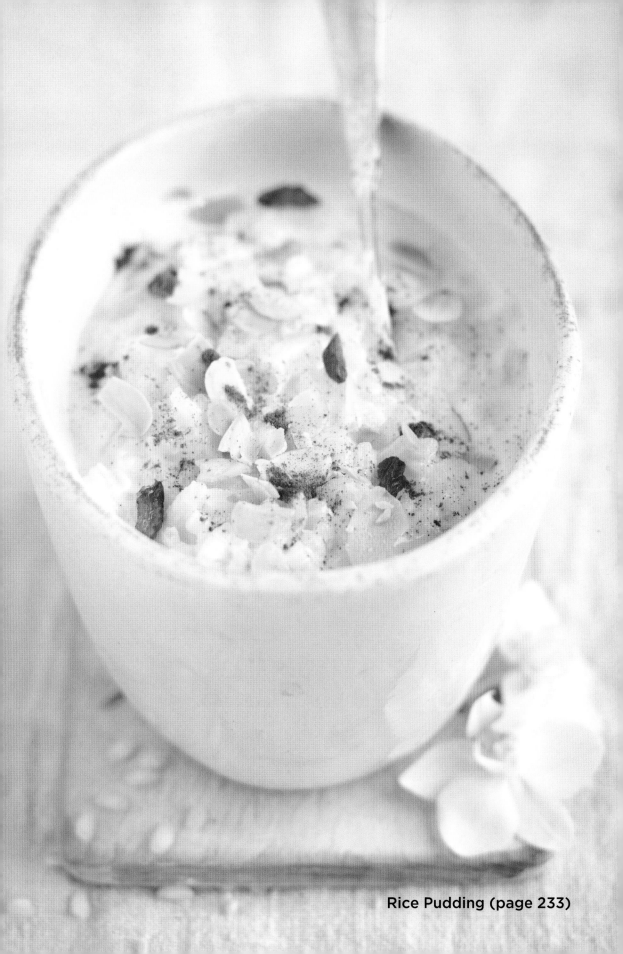

Rice Pudding (page 233)

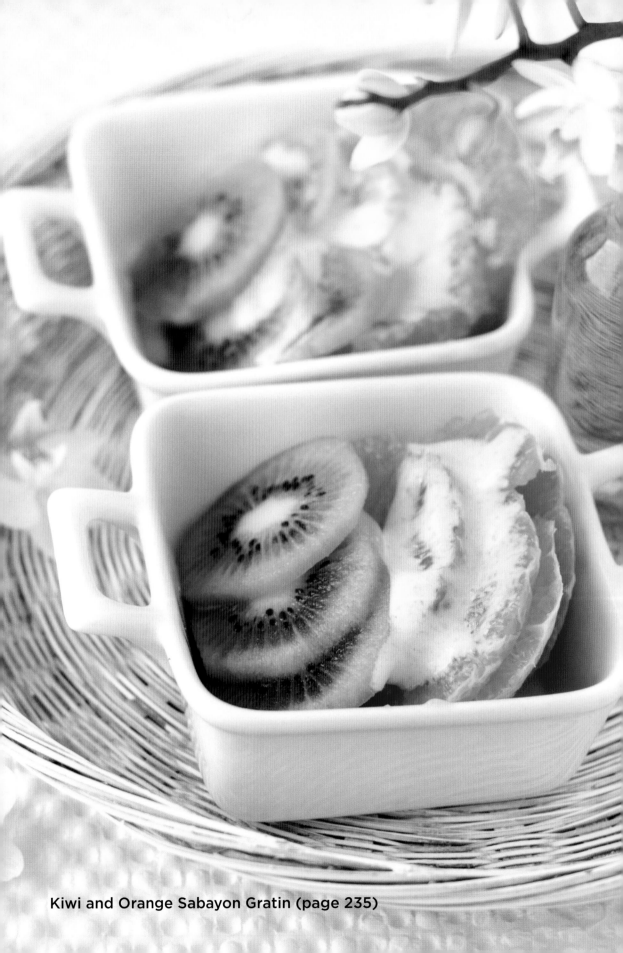

Kiwi and Orange Sabayon Gratin (page 235)

Provence-Style Chicken

Preparation time:

15 minutes

Marinating time:

3 hours

Cooking time:

50 minutes

- **Rimmed baking sheet or baking dish, lined with foil**

4	bone-in chicken leg quarters, skin removed (about 2 lbs, 6 oz/ 1.2 kg total)	4
2 tbsp	olive paste	30 mL
3 tbsp	olive oil	45 mL
1 tbsp	freshly squeezed lemon juice	15 mL
1 tbsp	Parsley Base (page 93)	15 mL
¼ tsp	cayenne pepper	1 mL
	Salt and freshly ground black pepper	
2 cups	mini tomatoes	500 mL
½ cup	black olives	125 mL
1 tbsp	extra virgin olive oil	15 mL

1. Put the chicken, olive paste, olive oil, lemon juice, Parsley Base and cayenne in a sealable plastic bag. Season with a little salt and pepper. Seal the bag and turn it to coat the chicken with the marinade. Chill in the refrigerator at least 3 hours or overnight.

2. Preheat the oven to 375°F (190°C).

3. Arrange the chicken pieces on the prepared baking sheet, discarding any excess marinade. Bake for 35 minutes in the middle of the oven.

4. Meanwhile, in a bowl, mix the mini tomatoes and olives with the extra virgin olive oil. Add them to the chicken and bake for an additional 15 minutes, until juices run clear when chicken is pierced. Serve.

NUTRIENTS PER SERVING	
Calories	300
Protein	30 g
Fat	18.0 g
Saturated fat	3.5 g
Carbohydrates	4 g
Fiber	2 g
Sodium	410 mg

Chicken Fajitas

**MAKES
4 SERVINGS**

Preparation time:

10 minutes

Marinating time:

8 hours

Cooking time:

20 minutes

A very tasty Mexican-American dish that is assembled at the table — always a kid pleaser.

3 tbsp	freshly squeezed lime juice	45 mL
2 tsp	ground cumin	10 mL
	Salt and freshly ground black pepper	
1	large boneless skinless chicken breast (14 oz/400 g)	1
2 tbsp	Garlic-Infused Oil (page 147)	30 mL
½	bulb fennel (6 oz/170 g), trimmed and thinly sliced	½
1	yellow or red bell pepper, cut into strips	1
8	6-inch (15 cm) corn tortillas (about 13 oz/360 g total)	8
¼ cup	lactose-free plain yogurt (optional)	60 mL

1. In a shallow dish, whisk together the lime juice, cumin, salt and pepper. Add the chicken, turning to coat well. Cover and chill in the refrigerator overnight.

2. Heat the Garlic-Infused Oil in a skillet over medium heat. Add the yellow pepper and fennel, then sauté for around 10 minutes, until the peppers are softened. Add salt and pepper. Set aside.

3. Preheat broiler or barbecue grill to medium.

4. Drain marinade from chicken breast, discarding marinade, and pat dry. Put it on the rack of a broiler pan and broil under a preheated broiler, 2½ to 4 inches (7 to 10 cm) from the heat, for about 5 to 6 minutes on each side or until no longer pink inside and a thermometer inserted in the thickest part registers 170°F (77°C). (Alternatively, place on preheated grill, and grill for 10 to 12 minutes total, turning once.)

NUTRIENTS PER SERVING

Calories	410
Protein	29 g
Fat	13.0 g
Saturated fat	2.0 g
Carbohydrates	48 g
Fiber	6 g
Sodium	80 mg

5. Transfer to a cutting board, then slice thinly and arrange the slices on a serving platter with the vegetables.

6. Meanwhile, stack up to 4 tortillas at a time in a microwave-safe plastic bag and microwave on High for 30 to 60 seconds or until they are heated through and pliable.

7. At the table, put a few slices of chicken on each tortilla and add some of the sautéed vegetables and yogurt (if using). Roll up the tortilla to enclose the filling. Enjoy.

Vegan Variation

Substitute firm regular tofu for chicken. Tofu can be marinated for a couple of hours instead of overnight.

Chicken Saltimbocca

Preparation time:

5 minutes

Cooking time:

10 minutes

This recipe is inspired by saltimbocca alla Romana, a classic Roman dish. In this version, the traditional veal cutlets are replaced with chicken breast cutlets.

TIP

Keep the serving plates in the oven at the lowest setting so they are warm when you serve.

	NUTRIENTS PER SERVING	
Calories	280
Protein	39 g
Fat	11.0 g
Saturated fat	2.0 g
Carbohydrates	5 g
Fiber	1 g
Sodium	300 mg

- **Preheat oven to 170°F (77°C)**
- **Meat mallet or rolling pin**

2	boneless skinless chicken breasts (about 1¼ lbs/600 g total)	2
2 tbsp	cornstarch	30 mL
12	fresh sage leaves	12
6	thin slices Parma ham or prosciutto (about 2⅓ oz/65 g total), cut in half	6
2 tbsp	olive oil	30 mL
3 tbsp	white wine	45 mL
	Salt and freshly ground black pepper	
⅓ cup	Allergen-Free Vegetable Broth (page 116)	75 mL
4 tsp	non-hydrogenated margarine	20 mL

1. Slice the chicken breasts horizontally into 12 very thin cutlets. Flatten these cutlets using a meat mallet or rolling pin. Coat each cutlet with the cornstarch; then shake off the excess.

2. Place a leaf of sage on each piece of chicken and cover with a slice of prosciutto. Use a toothpick to keep the small sandwich together.

3. Heat the oil in a large skillet. Working in batches, add a few cutlets at a time. Start with the chicken side down, and cook over high heat. After 3 minutes, turn the cutlet to brown the prosciutto side. Deglaze with some of the wine. Lower the heat, cover and cook for 2 minutes. Season with a pinch of salt (prosciutto is already fairly salty) and pepper to taste. Transfer the cutlets to a plate, cover with foil and keep them warm in the oven. Repeat with the remaining cutlets.

4. Pour the broth into the pan and cook over high heat until reduced by half, about 1 minute. Remove the pan from the heat, then stir in the margarine until a sauce consistency is obtained, about 30 seconds.

5. Place the cutlets on warmed plates, remove the toothpicks, spoon the sauce over the cutlets and serve.

Blue Cheese Turkey Burgers

Preparation time:

10 minutes

Cooking time:

10 minutes

A variation on the traditional cheeseburger, this recipe contains a creamy filling of melted blue cheese.

TIP
The FODMAP content of celery is borderline, so be sure to use the precise weight indicated in the recipe.

NUTRIENTS PER SERVING

Calories	380
Protein	30 g
Fat	15.0 g
Saturated fat	4.5 g
Carbohydrates	31 g
Fiber	5 g
Sodium	530 mg

- Preheat lightly oiled barbecue grill to medium (optional)

1	stalk celery (1⅓ oz/70 g)	1
1 lb	lean ground turkey or chicken	460 g
1½ tsp	dried oregano	7 mL
2 tsp	Dijon mustard	10 mL
	Salt and freshly ground black pepper	
1½ oz	blue cheese	40 g
8	slices gluten-free bread (about 13 oz/360 g total)	8
2 tsp	canola oil	10 mL
2 tsp	ketchup (optional)	10 mL
2 tsp	Dijon mustard (optional)	10 mL
	Tomato slices and lettuce leaves (optional)	

1. Coarsely chop the celery and put it in a bowl. Add the ground turkey, oregano, mustard, salt and pepper. Mix well using a fork, then bring the combined ingredients together with your hands to form a firm mixture.

2. Divide the mixture into 8 portions. Shape each portion into rounds and flatten each one slightly. Crumble the cheese and place a small amount in the center of 4 of the rounds. Place the remaining meat rounds on top of the cheese topped rounds. Use your hands to mold the rounds together, encasing the crumbled cheese and shaping them into burgers.

3. Grill the burgers, turning them once, for about 10 minutes or until a thermometer inserted in the center registers 165°F (74°C). (Alternatively, you may cook the burgers in a nonstick, heavy-bottomed pan, over very high heat on the stovetop.)

4. Place each burger in between 2 slices of bread. Serve with ketchup and mustard on the side, if using, adding a slice of tomato and lettuce, if desired.

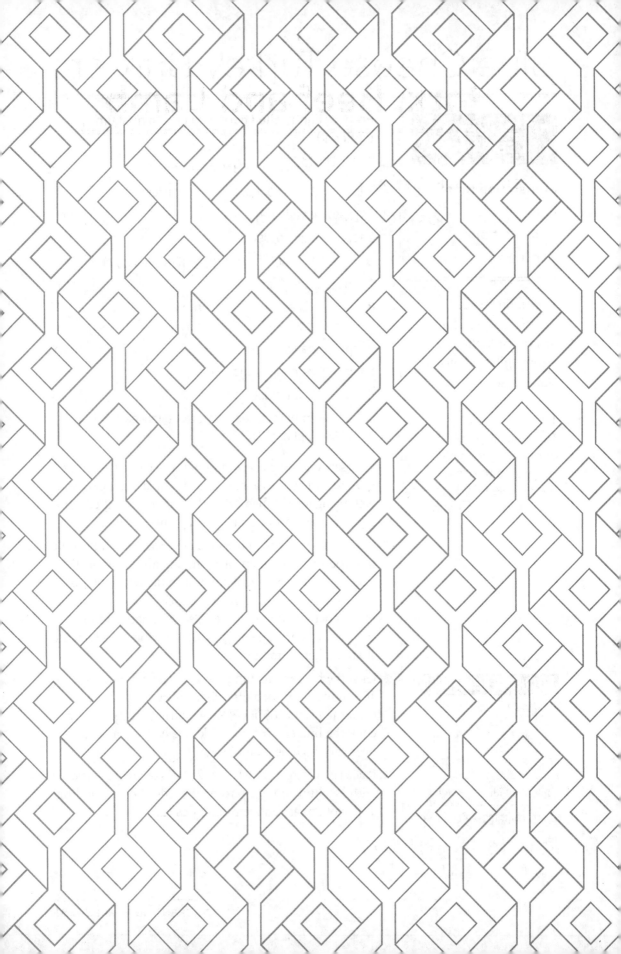

Pork, Beef and Lamb

Slow Cooker Ham with Beer and Maple Syrup

Preparation time:

10 minutes

Cooking time:

10 hours

Even though beer is made from barley or wheat, which do contain FODMAPs, it is in fact a low-FODMAP drink. If you are following a gluten-free diet, make sure to choose a gluten-free beer.

- Minimum 4-quart slow cooker

1½ lbs	boneless smoked ham, rind removed	700 g
1½ tsp	dry mustard	7 mL
⅔ cup	beer, preferably lager	150 mL
¼ cup	pure maple syrup	60 mL
	Freshly ground black pepper	

1. Put the ham in a large pot and cover with cold water. Bring to a boil, then simmer for 10 minutes. (This optional step reduces the saltiness of the ham.) Drain well.

2. Transfer the ham to the slow cooker stoneware and add the mustard, beer and maple syrup. Cover and cook on High for 7 to 8 hours, or on Low for 10 to 12 hours, until the meat is so tender that it falls apart when you insert a fork. Add a little pepper, then serve.

NUTRIENTS PER SERVING	
Calories	230
Protein	29 g
Fat	8.0 g
Saturated fat	2.5 g
Carbohydrates	4 g
Fiber	0 g
Sodium	1330 mg

Pork Chops with a Mustard Sauce

MAKES 4 SERVINGS

Preparation time:

5 minutes

Cooking time:

15 minutes

TIP

Keep the individual serving plates in the oven at the lowest setting so they are warm when you serve.

• **Preheat oven to 170°F (77°C)**

4	bone-in pork loin chops, about ¾-inch (2 cm) thick (about 1½ lbs/700 g total)	4
½ tsp	freshly ground black pepper	2 mL
2 tbsp	canola oil	30 mL
1 tbsp	Garlic-Infused Oil (page 147)	15 mL
½ cup	Allergen-Free Vegetable Broth (page 116)	125 mL
2 tbsp	Dijon mustard	30 mL
3 tbsp	lactose-free heavy or whipping (35%) cream	45 mL
2 tsp	freshly squeezed lemon juice	10 mL
	Salt	

1. Pat the pork chops dry, then sprinkle with pepper. Set aside.

2. Heat a dry, heavy skillet over medium-high heat. When the skillet is hot, add the canola oil, swirling the pan to coat the bottom, then add the chops and brown for 2 minutes on each side. Transfer the pork chops to a plate, then set them in the oven, loosely covered with foil, to keep warm.

3. Meanwhile, add the Garlic-Infused Oil to the skillet. Add the broth and boil for 2 minutes, scraping up any brown bits. Add the mustard and cream, return the mixture to a boil, then add the lemon juice. Return the pork chops to the skillet. Simmer, uncovered, until the sauce is slightly thickened and just a hint of pink remains in pork, 3 to 4 minutes. Add salt to taste. Serve on warmed plates.

NUTRIENTS PER SERVING

Calories	300
Protein	26 g
Fat	20.0 g
Saturated fat	6.0 g
Carbohydrates	3 g
Fiber	1 g
Sodium	210 mg

Prosciutto-Wrapped Pork Tenderloin

**MAKES
4 SERVINGS**

• **MAKE AHEAD** •

Preparation time:

10 minutes

Cooking time:

25 minutes

Standing time:

10 minutes

A quick and simple weeknight meal that looks like a showy weekend meal and tastes just wonderful.

NUTRIENTS PER SERVING	
Calories	230
Protein	41 g
Fat	7.0 g
Saturated fat	2.0 g
Carbohydrates	1 g
Fiber	0 g
Sodium	600 mg

• **Preheat oven to 425°F (220°C)**
• **Roasting pan**

2	small pork tenderloins (about 1¼ lbs/600 g total)	2
¼ tsp	salt	1 mL
¼ tsp	freshly ground black pepper	1 mL
12	thin slices prosciutto (about 4½ oz/130 g total)	12
10	fresh sage leaves	10
1 tbsp	olive oil	15 mL
	Hot water	

1. Pat the pork tenderloins dry and sprinkle all over with salt and pepper. Divide up the prosciutto slices and sage leaves equally to wrap the two tenderloins. Wrap one at a time. On a work surface, lay out the prosciutto slices lengthwise, extending away from you, and with a slight overlap along the sides. Scatter the sage leaves crosswise on top. Put one pork tenderloin on top of the sage, across the middle of the prosciutto "sheet," tucking the end of the tenderloin underneath if very thin, for more uniform cooking. Wrap the prosciutto around the meat to enclose it. Wrap the second tenderloin in the same manner.

The cooled pork can be stored in an airtight container in the refrigerator for up to 3 days. Reheat in the microwave before serving.

Keep the serving plates warm on the stove while you're preparing the dish.

2. Place both wrapped tenderloins, seam side down, in the roasting pan, spacing them at least 2 inches (5 cm) apart. Brush the prosciutto all over with oil. Roast the pork tenderloins in the middle of the preheated oven until a thermometer inserted in the center of the meat reaches 150°F (66°C). Pork is at its best when slightly "pink": as a reference only, you may estimate a cooking time of about 25 minutes for a tenderloin weighing 1 lb (450 g), or about 22 minutes for a 10 ½ oz (300 g) tenderloin (the exact cooking time depends on the actual temperature of your oven and the tenderloin size).

3. When the meat is done, take it out of the oven, cover it loosely with foil and let stand for 5 to 10 minutes before slicing, to allow the juices to distribute evenly.

4. Meanwhile, pour a few teaspoons (10 to 15 mL) of hot water in the roasting pan to dilute the meat drippings, then spoon this sauce over the pork slices. Serve on warmed plates.

Slow Cooker Pulled Pork

Preparation time:

5 minutes

Cooking time:

8 hours

This can be savored in a sandwich or as a main course with vegetables.

TIP

Tomato passata is a purée of raw tomatoes that have been peeled and seeded. If you cannot find it at your supermarket, look for it at specialty Italian grocery stores.

NUTRIENTS PER SERVING	
Calories	280
Protein	23 g
Fat	12.0 g
Saturated fat	3.5 g
Carbohydrates	22 g
Fiber	1 g
Sodium	200 mg

4 tsp	Garlic-Infused Oil (page 147)	20 mL
½	bulb fennel (6 oz/170 g), trimmed and finely chopped (see tip, page 199)	½
⅔ cup	tomato passata (see tip)	150 mL
¼ cup	apple cider vinegar	60 mL
¼ cup	maple jelly (or 2 tbsp/30 mL pure maple syrup)	60 mL
2½ tsp	packed brown sugar	12 mL
2 tsp	Worcestershire sauce	10 mL
¼ tsp	hot pepper sauce, such as Tabasco	1 mL
2 tsp	Dijon mustard	10 mL
¾ tsp	dried oregano	3 mL
⅛ tsp	cayenne pepper	0.5 mL
	Salt	
1¾ lb	boneless pork shoulder blade (butt) roast, without rind, fat trimmed off	800 g
	Freshly ground black pepper	

1. Heat the Garlic-Infused Oil in a pan over medium heat. Add the fennel and sauté until softened, about 3 minutes. Transfer to the slow cooker stoneware. Add the tomato passata, vinegar, maple jelly, brown sugar, Worcestershire sauce, hot pepper sauce, mustard, oregano and cayenne pepper. Mix well to combine. Add a pinch of salt.

2. Add the pork and stir to coat it with the sauce. Cover and cook on Low for 8 hours or until fork-tender.

3. Take the meat out of the pot and pull it apart with a fork. If necessary, reduce the sauce in a small saucepan and add it to the meat. Adjust the seasoning, then serve.

Bacon, Lettuce and Tomato Penne

Preparation time:

10 minutes

Cooking time:

15 minutes

TIP

Keep the serving plates warm on the stove while you're preparing the dish.

- **Preheat oven to 450°F (230°C)**
- **Small baking dish**

3 cups	mini tomatoes	750 mL
2 tbsp	olive oil	30 mL
4	slices bacon (2¾ oz/80 g total), chopped	4
1	bunch arugula (5 oz/150 g)	1
4 cups	gluten-free penne pasta (11 oz/320 g)	1 L
	Salt	
3½ oz	feta cheese, crumbled	100 g
	Freshly ground black pepper	
4 tsp	grated Parmesan cheese (optional)	20 mL

1. Place the tomatoes in the baking dish. Pour in the oil, then coat the tomatoes thoroughly and spread into a single layer. Bake in preheated oven for 5 to 7 minutes, until the skins split open.

2. Sauté the bacon pieces in a nonstick skillet over medium heat until they are crispy, then drain them on a paper towel. Reserve skillet.

3. Rinse and dry the arugula, remove and discard the stems, then set the leaves aside.

4. Meanwhile, cook the penne in a large pot of salted boiling water until al dente. Drain.

5. Transfer the baked tomatoes and juices to the skillet, add the crumbled feta cheese and put the bacon pieces back into the pan. Pour the drained penne into the pan, add the arugula and toss well. Add pepper to taste and grated Parmesan (if desired). Serve in warmed dishes.

NUTRIENTS PER SERVING

Calories	440
Protein	14 g
Fat	14.0 g
Saturated fat	5.0 g
Carbohydrates	63 g
Fiber	4 g
Sodium	420 mg

Spaghetti Carbonara

Preparation time:

10 minutes

Cooking time:

10 minutes

The name "carbonara" comes from the Italian carbone, meaning "coal" or "charcoal," and some believe it was created by those who extracted coal from the mines in the Latium region (near Rome).

TIP

Keep the serving dishes in the oven at the lowest setting so they are warm when you serve.

- **Preheat oven to 170°F (77°C)**
- **Large ovenproof serving bowl**

11 oz	gluten-free spaghetti	320 g
	Salt	
6	slices bacon or pancetta (4 oz/120 g total), chopped	6
2	large eggs	2
	Freshly ground black pepper	
2 tbsp	unsalted butter	30 mL
2 tbsp	grated Parmesan cheese	30 mL

1. Cook the spaghetti in a large pot of salted boiling water until al dente.

2. Fry the bacon in a nonstick skillet until the bacon is crisp. Set the bacon aside on a paper towel to drain the excess fat.

3. Whisk the eggs in the ovenproof serving bowl, add salt and pepper, then beat for 1 minute with a fork. Set the bowl aside in the preheated oven to keep it warm.

4. Drain the spaghetti and immediately pour it into the serving bowl. Mix rapidly to cook the eggs and coat the spaghetti at the same time. Add the fried bacon, the butter and the grated cheese. Adjust the seasoning before serving in warmed dishes.

NUTRIENTS PER SERVING	
Calories	430
Protein	15 g
Fat	13.0 g
Saturated fat	6.0 g
Carbohydrates	59 g
Fiber	3 g
Sodium	250 mg

Spicy Island Ribs

· MAKE AHEAD ·

Preparation time:

5 minutes

Marinating time:

8 hours

Cooking time:

1 hour 5 minutes

TIP

Instead of grilling the ribs you can bake them. Preheat the oven to 350°F (180°C). Place the ribs on a baking sheet. Bake for about 25 minutes, adding a few tablespoons (30 to 45 mL) of marinade as needed. Serve.

3 lbs	pork back or side ribs	1.5 kg
	Water	
2 tbsp	Dijon mustard	30 mL
2 tbsp	soy sauce	30 mL
¼ cup	pure maple syrup	60 mL
1 tbsp	white vinegar	15 mL
2 tsp	Worcestershire sauce	10 mL
¾ tsp	hot pepper sauce, such as Tabasco	3 mL

1. Place the ribs in a large pot, cover with water, bring to a boil, then reduce the heat and simmer, covered, for 45 minutes. Remove the ribs and drain.

2. In a shallow dish, mix the Dijon mustard, soy sauce, maple syrup, vinegar, Worcestershire sauce and hot pepper sauce. Add the ribs, turning them to coat well. Cover and chill in the refrigerator overnight or up to 48 hours.

3. Preheat barbecue grill to high.

4. Place the ribs on the hot grill, reserving the marinade, and cook for about 10 to 12 minutes on each side, brushing them with more marinade as needed.

NUTRIENTS PER SERVING	
Calories	380
Protein	47 g
Fat	13.0 g
Saturated fat	5.0 g
Carbohydrates	16 g
Fiber	0 g
Sodium	310 mg

Steak, Pepper and Bok Choy Stir-Fry

**MAKES
4 SERVINGS**

• MAKE AHEAD •

• FREEZABLE •

Preparation time:

10 minutes

Marinating time:

1 hour

Cooking time:

20 minutes

	• Ovenproof serving dish	
14 oz	beef strip loin steak(s)	400 g
¼ cup	soy sauce	60 mL
4 tsp	unseasoned pure tomato paste	20 mL
3 tbsp	cornstarch	45 mL
2 tsp	granulated sugar	10 mL
1 tbsp	grated gingerroot, divided	15 mL
3 tbsp	Garlic-Infused Oil (page 147), divided	45 mL
½	bulb fennel (6 oz/170 g), trimmed and coarsely chopped	½
2	yellow or red bell peppers, cut into strips	2
1	dried chile pepper, minced	1
	Salt	
4	small bok choy, quartered or halved (1¾ lbs/800 g total)	4
	Freshly ground black pepper	

1. Slice the meat into strips ¼- to ½-inch (0.5 to 1 cm) wide and about 2 inches (5 cm) long. Mix with the soy sauce, tomato paste, cornstarch, sugar and a bit of grated ginger. Chill for at least an hour in the refrigerator.

2. Preheat the oven to the lowest setting, approximately 170°F (77°C). Put a serving dish in the oven.

NUTRIENTS PER SERVING	
Calories	330
Protein	24 g
Fat	19.0 g
Saturated fat	4.0 g
Carbohydrates	19 g
Fiber	4 g
Sodium	750 mg

The FODMAP content of tomato paste and fennel is borderline, so be sure to use the precise volume or weight indicated in the recipe.

The cooled stir-fry can be stored in an airtight container in the refrigerator for up to 3 days. Reheat in the microwave before serving.

3. Heat $\frac{1}{2}$ to 1 tbsp (7 to 15 mL) Garlic-Infused Oil in a skillet or wok over medium-high heat. Add the fennel, bell pepper and chile pepper. Add a little salt and stir-fry for about 5 minutes, until they start to soften. Add the bok choy and stir-fry for 4 to 5 minutes, until cooked but still crunchy. Set the vegetables aside on the warmed serving dish in the oven.

4. Add the remaining Garlic-Infused Oil and the marinated meat. Reserve the remaining marinade. Stir-fry over medium heat for 5 to 7 minutes, until the meat is almost cooked. Put the vegetables back into the wok and add the remaining grated ginger. Stir in the reserved marinade. Cook, stirring, for another 2 minutes, ensuring marinade comes to a boil for at least 1 minute. Add salt and pepper to taste. Serve.

Vegan Variation

Regular firm tofu may be substituted for beef.

Thai Noodles with Beef

VEGAN OPTION

• MAKE AHEAD •

Preparation time:

15 minutes

Marinating time:

1 hour

Cooking time:

10 minutes

Standing time:

5 minutes

A simple, bright and colorful salad that's a meal in itself.

3 tbsp	freshly squeezed lime juice	45 mL
1½ tbsp	fish sauce	22 mL
4 tsp	canola oil	20 mL
4 tsp	granulated sugar	20 mL
1	dried chile pepper, finely chopped	1
14 oz	boneless beef top sirloin steak	400 g
4 oz	rice stick noodles	120 g
1 cup	broccoli florets	250 mL
1	carrot, grated	1
1⅓ cups	bean sprouts	325 mL
2 tbsp	finely chopped fresh mint	30 mL

1. Put the lime juice, fish sauce, oil, sugar and chile pepper in a small bowl and whisk well. Take 1 to 2 tbsp (15 to 30 mL) and pour it into a shallow dish, setting aside the rest. Add the steak to the shallow dish, then turn it to coat well. Cover, put it in the refrigerator and let it marinate for 1 hour.

2. Cook the rice stick noodles in a large pot of salted boiling water for about 3 minutes or according to package directions, until al dente. Drain and put them in a salad bowl.

3. Blanch the broccoli in salted boiling water until tender-crisp, about 4 minutes. Drain well and add it to the salad bowl.

4. Add the carrot, bean sprouts and mint to the salad bowl, pour the reserved dressing over the salad and toss well.

NUTRIENTS PER SERVING	
Calories	370
Protein	27 g
Fat	13.0 g
Saturated fat	3.5 g
Carbohydrates	36 g
Fiber	2 g
Sodium	520 mg

5. Preheat the barbecue grill to medium-high.

6. Put the steak on a warm grill and cook for about 3 minutes per side, turning once, for medium-rare. (Alternatively, cook the steak in a heavy-bottomed skillet on the stovetop.)

7. Transfer the steak to a cutting board and let it stand for 5 minutes to reabsorb the juices. Slice thinly across the grain and on a diagonal bias.

8. Arrange the steak slices on the noodle salad, then serve.

Vegan Variation

Omit the fish sauce and swap the beef for tempeh.

Filet Mignon with a Creamy Paprika Sauce

Preparation time:

5 minutes

Cooking time:

10 minutes

Standing time:

10 minutes

TIPS

For proper cooking all the way through, it is important to let the beef stand at room temperature for 30 minutes before cooking.

Keep the serving plates in the oven at the lowest setting so they are warm when you serve.

NUTRIENTS PER SERVING	
Calories	310
Protein	28 g
Fat	19.0 g
Saturated fat	7.0 g
Carbohydrates	5 g
Fiber	1 g
Sodium	270 mg

4	beef tenderloin medallions, each about ³⁄₄-inch (2 cm) thick (about 1¼ lbs/600 g total)	4
	Salt and freshly ground black pepper	
3 tbsp	Garlic-Infused Oil (page 147)	45 mL
½ cup	Allergen-Free Vegetable Broth (page 116)	125 mL
1 tbsp	paprika	15 mL
2 tbsp	Dijon mustard	30 mL
4 tsp	Worcestershire sauce	20 mL
¼ cup	lactose-free heavy or whipping (35%) cream	60 mL

1. Pat the beef dry and sprinkle with a little bit of salt and pepper.

2. Heat the Garlic-Infused Oil in a heavy skillet over medium heat until hot but not smoking. Add the beef and cook for about 4 minutes on each side for medium-rare, turning once. Transfer to a cutting board and let stand, loosely covered with foil, for 10 minutes to reabsorb the juices.

3. Meanwhile, deglaze the skillet with the broth, scraping up brown bits. Bring to a boil and cook for 1 minute. Reduce the heat, then add the paprika and cook for 2 minutes, stirring. Whisk in the mustard, Worcestershire sauce, lactose-free cream, and any beef juice from the cutting board. Bring just to a simmer and cook for 1 minute. Add salt and pepper to taste. Thin the sauce with a few tablespoons (30 to 45 mL) of water, if necessary.

4. Serve beef on warmed plates, with the sauce spooned on top.

Asian Beef and Vegetable Soup

MAKES 4 SERVINGS

Preparation time:
10 minutes

Cooking time:
10 minutes

1 tbsp	Garlic-Infused Oil (page 147)	15 mL
1 tbsp	grated gingerroot	15 mL
1	dried chile pepper, minced	1
3 cups	Allergen-Free Vegetable Broth (page 116)	750 mL
3 cups	water	750 mL
2 tbsp	fish sauce	30 mL
	Freshly ground black pepper	
11 oz	very thinly sliced beef for hot pot (Chinese fondue)	320 g
5½ oz	rice stick noodles	160 g
2	carrots, grated	2
2¾ cups	bean sprouts (7 oz/200 g)	675 mL

1. Heat the Garlic-Infused Oil in a saucepan over medium-low heat. Add the ginger and chile pepper. Sauté for 3 minutes. Pour in the broth and water. Stir in the fish sauce and a little pepper. Bring to a boil, then lower the heat and simmer for a few minutes. Adjust the seasoning. Add the meat slices, warm up the meat broth for 1 minute, then take the saucepan off the heat.

2. Meanwhile, cook the rice sticks for about 4 minutes in a large pot of salted boiling water or according to package directions. Drain in a colander, then rinse and drain again. Set aside.

3. Portion out the carrots into four individual serving bowls, each at least 2-cup (500 mL) capacity. Add the bean sprouts and cooked rice noodles. Pour in the hot broth and serve.

Vegan Variation

Swap out the beef for tofu and omit the fish sauce. To give the tofu more flavor, marinate it in a few tablespoons (30 to 45 mL) of soy sauce and sesame oil for a few minutes before sautéing in a hot pan then adding it to the soup.

NUTRIENTS PER SERVING

Calories	420
Protein	29 g
Fat	14.0 g
Saturated fat	3.0 g
Carbohydrates	49 g
Fiber	5 g
Sodium	940 mg

Flemish Beef Stew

• MAKE AHEAD •

• FREEZABLE •

Preparation time:

15 minutes

Cooking time:

2½ hours

This is the national Belgian dish. In some regions, bread spread with mustard is added toward the end of the cooking to give a special texture to the sauce. Rodenbach red beer is traditionally used in this recipe, but any good red beer (from Belgium, if possible) will do.

- **Preheat oven to 325°F (160°C)**
- **Stovetop-safe and ovenproof Dutch oven, casserole dish or large pot**

1¾ lb	boneless beef blade pot roast	800 g
	Salt and freshly ground black pepper	
2 tbsp	canola oil	30 mL
½	bulb fennel (6 oz/170 g), trimmed and finely chopped	½
2 tbsp	cornstarch	30 mL
1⅓ cups	beer	325 mL
2	bay leaves	2
1	sprig fresh rosemary	1
1½ tsp	packed brown sugar	7 mL
1½ tsp	wine vinegar	7 mL
	Water (optional)	
1	rutabaga or turnip (5 oz/150 g)	1
2	potatoes (14 oz/400 g total)	2

1. Cut the beef into large cubes, about 1⅔ inches (4 cm), and sprinkle with salt and pepper.
2. Heat the oil in the Dutch oven over high heat. Add the beef cubes in batches, turning them until dark brown on all sides, 7 to 10 minutes. Take the meat out of the pot using a slotted spoon, then transfer to a plate.

NUTRIENTS PER SERVING	
Calories	370
Protein	27 g
Fat	13.0 g
Saturated fat	3.5 g
Carbohydrates	29 g
Fiber	3 g
Sodium	75 mg

TIP

The FODMAP content of fennel is borderline, so be sure to use the precise weight indicated in the recipe.

3. Add the fennel to the pot and sauté over medium heat for about 5 minutes, then add the cornstarch and cook for 1 to 2 minutes, stirring. Pour in the beer, then return the meat to the pot and stir. Add the bay leaves, rosemary, brown sugar and vinegar. Pour in some water if necessary to cover the meat.

4. Cover and bake in the middle of the preheated oven for 2 hours, until the meat is tender.

5. Meanwhile, peel the turnip and potatoes and cut them into large chunks, then add them to the stew. Pour in some warm water if too dry. Season with salt, cover and continue to bake for an additional 20 to 25 minutes, until the vegetables are tender. Serve.

Beef Stew en Papillote

· MAKE AHEAD ·

· FREEZABLE ·

Preparation time:

10 minutes

Cooking time:

3 hours

This slow-cooking method — in which beef is wrapped in foil, requires no supervision and creates no mess — is ideal for less tender and less expensive cuts of meat. The final result: a welcoming aroma in the house and a juicy and tasty meal.

- **Preheat the oven to 275°F (135°C)**
- **Rimmed baking sheet**

¼ cup	ketchup	60 mL
1½ tsp	cornstarch	7 mL
1 tbsp	soy sauce	15 mL
¾ tsp	hot pepper sauce, such as Tabasco	3 mL
½ tsp	dry mustard	2 mL
2 lb	boneless beef blade pot roast	1 kg

1. In a small bowl, mix the ketchup, cornstarch, soy sauce, hot pepper sauce and mustard.

2. Put the pot roast on a large sheet of heavy-duty foil, spread the ketchup mixture on top, then wrap and seal thoroughly (you may want to add an additional sheet to ensure that the juices are well trapped inside).

3. Put the package on the baking sheet, then bake for 3 hours in the middle of the preheated oven, until beef is fork-tender. Serve the meat with its juices.

Variation

To cook in a slow cooker instead of the oven, reduce the ketchup to 2 tbsp (30 mL) and the soy sauce to 1½ tsp (7 mL), and add 2 tbsp (30 mL) water to the sauce. Instead of wrapping the pot roast in foil, place it in a minimum 4-quart slow cooker and spread the ketchup mixture on top. Cover and cook on Low for 7 hours or on High for 4 hours.

NUTRIENTS PER SERVING	
Calories	250
Protein	31 g
Fat	10.0 g
Saturated fat	4.0 g
Carbohydrates	6 g
Fiber	0 g
Sodium	190 mg

Beef and Vegetable Curry

Preparation time:

10 minutes

Cooking time:

35 minutes

TIPS

Keep the serving plates in the oven at the lowest setting so they are warm when you serve.

The cooled curry can be transferred to airtight containers and stored in the refrigerator for up to 3 days or in the freezer for up to 3 months. Thaw in the refrigerator overnight, if necessary. Reheat before serving.

NUTRIENTS PER SERVING	
Calories	390
Protein	27 g
Fat	19.0 g
Saturated fat	6.0 g
Carbohydrates	27 g
Fiber	5 g
Sodium	200 mg

2 tbsp	Garlic-Infused Oil (page 147)	30 mL
1 lb	lean ground beef	460 g
1½ tbsp	curry powder	22 mL
½ tsp	ground turmeric	2 mL
⅛ tsp	ground cinnamon	0.5 mL
⅛ tsp	cayenne pepper	0.5 mL
1 tsp	grated gingerroot	5 mL
2	potatoes (14 oz/400 g total), peeled and diced	2
1	carrot, peeled and diced	1
1⅔ cups	canned tomatoes, with juice	400 mL
	Water	
½ cup	frozen peas	125 mL
	Salt and freshly ground black pepper	

1. Heat the Garlic-Infused Oil in a sauté pan over medium heat. Add the meat. Cook for about 5 minutes, stirring occasionally with a wooden spoon, until the meat loses its pink color. Add the curry, turmeric, cinnamon, cayenne and ginger. Cook for 1 minute.

2. Add the potatoes, carrot, tomatoes and about ½ cup (125 mL) water. Mix well. Bring to a boil, then reduce the heat, cover and simmer, stirring occasionally, for 30 minutes, or until the potatoes are done. Add more water if necessary to maintain a moist environment.

3. Stir in the peas and cook for an additional 5 minutes. Adjust the seasoning and serve on warmed plates.

Swedish Meatballs

• MAKE AHEAD •

• FREEZABLE •

Preparation time:

30 minutes

Standing time:

1 hour

Cooking time:

30 minutes

Köttbullar (*meatballs*)
*is a Swedish dish
traditionally served with
boiled potatoes and a
lingonberry sauce (similar
to cranberry sauce).
The spice used here is
the berry of a pimiento
tree. It is aptly named
"allspice" because it
tastes like a combination
of spices, mostly cloves,
cinnamon and nutmeg.*

NUTRIENTS PER SERVING	
Calories	300
Protein	23 g
Fat	17.0 g
Saturated fat	6.0 g
Carbohydrates	12 g
Fiber	1 g
Sodium	340 mg

• **Rimmed baking sheet, lined with foil**

½	potato (3½ oz/100 g)	½
2 tsp	fresh Italian (flat-leaf) parsley leaves	10 mL
2 tsp	fresh dill sprigs	10 mL
1	large egg	1
14 oz	lean ground beef	400 g
1½ tbsp	water (approx.)	22 mL
¼ tsp	ground allspice	1 mL
¼ tsp	salt (or to taste)	1 mL
	Freshly ground black pepper	
2½ tbsp	packed brown sugar	37 mL
2 tbsp	Dijon mustard	30 mL
2 tsp	wine vinegar	10 mL
2 tsp	canola oil	10 mL
2 tsp	olive oil	10 mL

1. Peel the potato and boil in a saucepan of water until
   very tender, for 20 to 25 minutes. Drain well, then put
   it in a bowl and mash.

2. Mince the parsley and dill. Add half to the bowl with
   the potato and set the rest aside. Add the egg, ground
   beef, water, allspice, salt and pepper to the bowl. Using
   your hands, blend the mixture together until it is just
   combined well (do not overmix). Form the mixture into
   ¾- to 1¼-inch (2 to 3 cm) balls and arrange them on a
   baking sheet or tray. Cover and chill in the refrigerator
   for at least 1 hour or overnight to firm up the meat
   mixture.

TIP

If you shape these into smaller meatballs, they may be served as appetizers, with extra sauce for dipping.

3. Meanwhile, in a small bowl, whisk together the brown sugar, mustard, vinegar, canola oil and reserved parsley and dill until the brown sugar is dissolved and mixture is blended. Set aside.

4. Preheat oven to 350°F (180°C).

5. Heat the olive oil in a large pan over medium heat. Working in batches, add the meatballs and sauté until they are golden on all sides, about 5 minutes. Transfer the meatballs to the prepared baking sheet and brush them with the sauce. Cover loosely with foil.

6. Bake in the middle of the oven for 25 to 30 minutes. (Alternatively, thread the meatballs onto soaked bamboo skewers and cook on the oiled rack of a barbecue grill.)

7. Serve the meatballs with any remaining sauce on the side.

Pasta in a Bolognese Meat Sauce

Preparation time:

5 minutes

Cooking time:

15 minutes

When cooking a pasta dish, remember to set aside a little bit of the pasta cooking water. This will not only help loosen the sauce a bit, but the starch contained in the water will help the sauce to coat the pasta evenly.

TIP

Keep the serving plates in the oven at the lowest setting so they are warm when you serve.

NUTRIENTS PER SERVING	
Calories	430
Protein	17 g
Fat	11.0 g
Saturated fat	3.0 g
Carbohydrates	63 g
Fiber	4 g
Sodium	100 mg

4 cups	gluten-free penne pasta (11 oz/320 g)	1 L
1⅓ cup	Bolognese Meat Sauce (opposite)	325 mL
4 tsp	extra virgin olive oil	20 mL
¼ cup	grated Parmesan cheese (optional)	60 mL
	Salt and freshly ground black pepper	

1. Cook the penne in a large pot of salted boiling water until al dente. Drain, reserving some of the pasta cooking water.

2. Meanwhile, heat the meat sauce in a saucepan over low heat. Add about ¼ cup (60 mL) pasta cooking water to dilute the sauce a bit, and warm up for just a few minutes.

3. Put the drained penne back into the pasta cooking pot, add the sauce and olive oil, and mix well. Sprinkle with Parmesan cheese, if desired, and season with salt and pepper. Serve in warmed dishes.

Preparation time:

5 minutes

Cooking time:

1 hour, 20 minutes

Named after the sumptuous cooking style of Bologna, Italy, ragù Bolognese is a thick, full-bodied meat and vegetable sauce enhanced with wine and milk or cream. It is a versatile sauce that can be used over pasta, as a filling in lasagna or cannelloni and in many other ways.

TIPS

The FODMAP content of celery, fennel and tomato paste is borderline, so be sure to use the precise weights or volume indicated in the recipe.

The sauce can be stored for up to 1 week in the refrigerator or up to 2 months in the freezer.

Bolognese Meat Sauce

1	bulb fennel (12 oz/360 g), trimmed	1
1	carrot	1
1/2	stalk celery (1 oz/35 g)	1/2
1	slice bacon	1
1 1/2 tbsp	Garlic-Infused Oil (page 147)	22 mL
13 oz	lean ground beef	360 g
	Salt and freshly ground pepper	
1/3 cup	lactose-free milk	75 mL
1/3 cup	white wine	75 mL
1 cup	canned diced tomatoes, with juice	250 mL
2 tsp	unseasoned pure tomato paste	10 mL
1 tsp	dried oregano	5 mL

1. Finely chop the fennel, carrot, celery and bacon.

2. Heat the Garlic-Infused Oil in a saucepan over medium heat. Add the vegetables and bacon, and cook until softened, 5 to 6 minutes, with some stirring. Add the meat, then add salt and pepper to taste. Cook, stirring frequently and breaking up the meat with a spoon, until it loses its pink color and starts browning, about 7 to 8 minutes.

3. Raise the heat to high and add the milk. Cook, stirring frequently, until the liquid has evaporated, about 3 minutes. Add the wine, then cook, stirring frequently, until the wine has evaporated, about 3 minutes.

4. Stir in the diced tomatoes, tomato paste and oregano, then cover and simmer gently over low heat for at least 1 hour. Stir occasionally and add some water as needed to prevent the sauce from becoming too dry. Season with additional salt and pepper. It is important to simmer all the ingredients until the sauce is thick and the beef very tender.

Variation

This can also be made in a pressure cooker; cover and bring up to full pressure in step 4. Reduce the cooking time to 15 minutes from the time it starts to spatter.

Lamb Shanks with Potatoes

Preparation time:

10 minutes

Cooking time:

2 hours, 20 minutes

*The slow-cooked lamb
and potatoes, stewed
in the pan juices with
thyme and lemon, make
for an excellent dish.*

TIP

This dish may be made
ahead through step 2,
cooled, covered and
refrigerated for up
to 1 day. Reheat until
boiling, then proceed
with step 3.

NUTRIENTS PER SERVING	
Calories	500
Protein	46 g
Fat	16.0 g
Saturated fat	6.0 g
Carbohydrates	37 g
Fiber	5 g
Sodium	270 mg

- **Stovetop-safe large, deep casserole dish, Dutch oven
or pot, with lid**

1 tbsp	Garlic-Infused Oil (page 147)	15 mL
4	lamb shanks (about 3 lbs/1.4 kg total)	4
	Salt and freshly ground black pepper	
4	sprigs fresh thyme	4
$\frac{1}{3}$ cup	white wine	75 mL
2 cups	Allergen-Free Vegetable Broth (page 116)	500 mL
4	potatoes ($1\frac{3}{4}$ lbs/800 g total), peeled and cut into pieces	4
$\frac{1}{4}$ cup	freshly squeezed lemon juice	60 mL
	Fresh thyme leaves	

1. Heat the Garlic-Infused Oil in the casserole dish over
high heat. Add the lamb shanks and brown well, turning
them until colored on all sides, about 10 minutes. About
halfway through the browning, sprinkle the lamb with
salt and pepper, then add the thyme sprigs.

2. When the meat is nicely colored, deglaze with the wine.
Add the broth, then bring to a boil. Turn the heat down
to low and cover. Cook at a slow simmer until the lamb
is tender, about $1\frac{1}{2}$ hours or a little longer.

3. Add the potatoes, then cover again. Raise the heat if
necessary (the mixture should boil) and continue to
cook until the potatoes are just about tender, 30 to
40 minutes. If the stew is too thin, raise the heat to
high and uncover to boil off some of the liquid.

4. When the potatoes are tender, adjust the seasoning.
Stir in the lemon juice and garnish with a few thyme
leaves. Serve.

Mint-Marinated Lamb Chops

Preparation time:

10 minutes

Marinating time:

8 hours

Cooking time:

15 minutes

TIP

Fresh mint leaves can be kept for up to 10 days in the refrigerator if wrapped in damp paper towels and placed in a plastic bag. Extra bits may be frozen by chopping them up and putting them in an ice tray filled with water.

2 tbsp	finely chopped fresh mint	30 mL
2 tsp	black peppercorns, crushed	10 mL
3 tbsp	olive oil	45 mL
1/3 cup	red wine	75 mL
2 tsp	granulated sugar	10 mL
4	lamb loin chops (about 22 oz/ 650 g total)	4
	Salt	

1. In a medium bowl, combine mint, peppercorns, olive oil, red wine and sugar, then mix well: the marinade should have a thick consistency. Add the lamb chops, toss well and cover with plastic wrap. Place the bowl in the refrigerator to marinate overnight.

2. Preheat barbecue grill to medium or preheat broiler.

3. Cook the chops on a grill for about 10 minutes, basting with the marinade and turning them once. (When basting with marinade, add it early in the cooking process, and never in the last 5 minutes, to make sure the marinade is thoroughly cooked.) Alternatively, place chops on a broiler pan and broil. Season with salt, then serve.

NUTRIENTS PER SERVING	
Calories	160
Protein	19 g
Fat	8.0 g
Saturated fat	2.5 g
Carbohydrates	2 g
Fiber	0 g
Sodium	35 mg

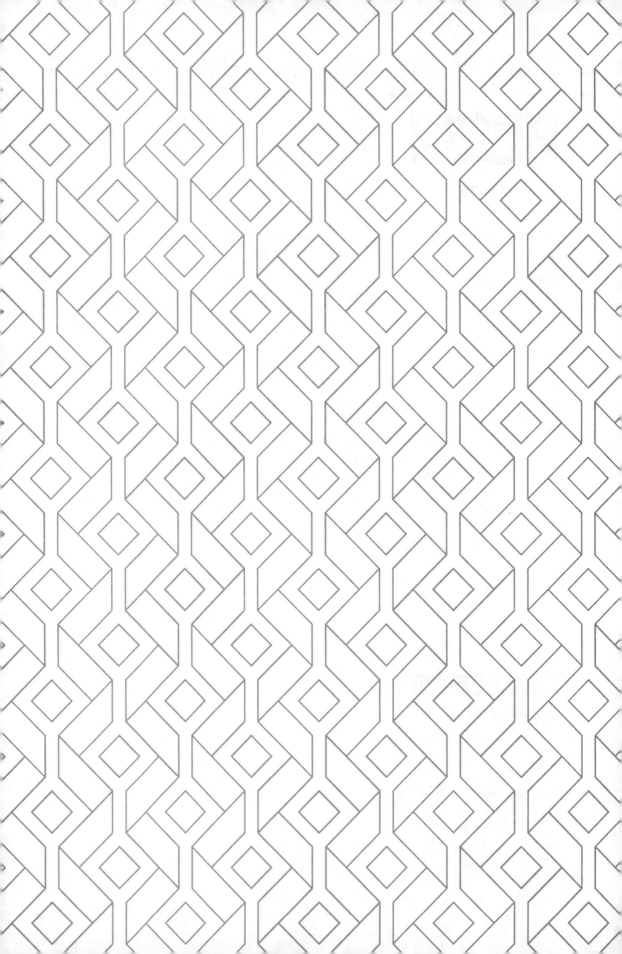

Side Dishes

Braised Bok Choy

**MAKES
4 SERVINGS**

Preparation time:

5 minutes

Cooking time:

10 minutes

Also called Chinese white cabbage, pak choy and white mustard cabbage, this member of the cabbage family is a mild, versatile vegetable with crunchy white stalks and tender dark green leaves. In the quantity specified in this recipe, bok choy is a great low-FODMAP green veggie choice.

4	small bok choy (1¾ lbs/800 g total)	4
¼ cup	non-hydrogenated margarine	60 mL
½ cup	Allergen-Free Vegetable Broth (page 116)	125 mL

1. Cut each bok choy in half lengthwise (or into quarters if large).
2. Heat the margarine in a large skillet over medium-high heat. Add the bok choy and sauté for 2 to 3 minutes, until they start coloring, then pour in the broth and cook, uncovered, for about 7 minutes, until the liquid is reduced and the bok choy is tender-crisp. Serve.

Vegan Variation

Substitute vegetable oil for the margarine.

NUTRIENTS PER SERVING

Calories	110
Protein	3 g
Fat	9.0 g
Saturated fat	1.5 g
Carbohydrates	5 g
Fiber	2 g
Sodium	160 mg

Sautéed Carrots

MAKES 4 SERVINGS

• MAKE AHEAD •

• FREEZABLE •

Preparation time:

7 minutes

Cooking time:

25 minutes

Make sure to have at least one portion of an orange vegetable each day.

TIP

The cooled carrots can be stored in an airtight container in the refrigerator for up to 3 days or in the freezer for up to 1 month. Thaw in the refrigerator if necessary, and reheat in the microwave before serving.

NUTRIENTS PER SERVING	
Calories	90
Protein	1 g
Fat	4.5 g
Saturated fat	0.5 g
Carbohydrates	13 g
Fiber	3 g
Sodium	95 mg

6	carrots (1¼ lbs/600 g total)	6
2 tbsp	non-hydrogenated margarine	30 mL
	Salt	

1. Peel and slice the carrots into thin rounds.

2. Heat the margarine in a pan over medium heat. Add the carrots. Cook for 5 minutes, uncovered, stirring frequently.

3. Add salt, cover and cook on low heat for about 20 minutes or until the carrots are soft.

Vegan Variation

Substitute vegetable oil for the margarine.

Skillet Endive

MAKES
4 SERVINGS

· MAKE AHEAD ·

Preparation time:

5 minutes

Cooking time:

30 minutes

TIP

The endive can be stored in the refrigerator for up to 3 days, then reheated before serving.

2 tbsp	olive oil	30 mL
4	Belgian endive (1¼ lbs/600 g total)	4
½ tsp	granulated sugar	2 mL
	Salt	

1. Heat the oil in a skillet over low heat. Add the endive. Add the sugar and salt to taste, then cover and cook over very low heat, turning the heads of endive occasionally, until they are very tender and caramelized all over, about 30 minutes.

2. Remove the lid and cook over high heat just long enough to evaporate some of the excess liquid. Serve with the juices.

NUTRIENTS PER SERVING

Calories	60
Protein	1 g
Fat	5.0 g
Saturated fat	0.5 g
Carbohydrates	5 g
Fiber	4 g
Sodium	3 mg

Okra with Tomatoes

MAKES 4 SERVINGS

· **MAKE AHEAD** ·

· **FREEZABLE** ·

Preparation time:

10 minutes

Cooking time:

15 minutes

Okra can be found year-round in ethnic groceries and supermarkets. It contains lots of soluble fiber, which can help relieve constipation and diarrhea.

TIP

The okra can be stored in the refrigerator for up to 3 days or frozen for up to 3 months; thaw, if necessary, before reheating.

NUTRIENTS PER SERVING	
Calories	50
Protein	1 g
Fat	4.0 g
Saturated fat	0.5 g
Carbohydrates	5 g
Fiber	2 g
Sodium	45 mg

4 tsp	Garlic-Infused Oil (page 147)	20 mL
1/2	green bell pepper, chopped	1/2
7 oz	whole okra, ends trimmed	200 g
1/2	dried chile pepper, minced	1/2
2/3 cup	canned diced tomatoes, with juice	150 mL
4 tsp	freshly squeezed lemon juice	20 mL
	Salt and freshly ground black pepper	

1. Heat the Garlic-Infused Oil in a skillet over medium heat. Add the green pepper, okra and chile pepper, and cook for 3 minutes, with occasional stirring.

2. Stir in the tomatoes and lemon juice. Bring the mixture to a boil, then reduce the heat, cover and simmer for about 10 minutes, until the okra is tender. Adjust the seasoning and serve.

Oven-Roasted Peppers

VEGAN

· MAKE AHEAD ·

· FREEZABLE ·

Preparation time:

5 minutes

Cooking time:

30 minutes

Standing time:

45 to 50 minutes

Peppers may be either roasted or grilled, the choice being a matter of personal preference: roasting takes longer but yields peppers that are more fully cooked, hence easier to digest and to purée than those that are grilled. Grilling is quicker and yields firmer peppers.

NUTRIENTS PER SERVING	
Calories	70
Protein	1 g
Fat	3.5 g
Saturated fat	0.5 g
Carbohydrates	11 g
Fiber	2 g
Sodium	4 mg

- Preheat the oven to 425°F (220°C)
- Baking dish or roasting pan

4	yellow or red bell peppers ($1^3/_4$ lbs/800 g total)	4
4 tsp	extra virgin olive oil	20 mL
	Salt and freshly ground black pepper	
	Extra virgin olive oil	

1. Clean the peppers with a wet towel, pat dry, and place in the baking dish or roasting pan. Cook in the middle of the preheated oven for about 30 minutes or until peppers are soft and browned in spots. Turn them twice during cooking.

2. Remove from oven, cover or wrap in a paper bag and let cool down for about 15 to 20 minutes (the moisture kept in the bag or under the cover will help the peeling). Remove the stem. Peel and cut each pepper lengthwise into 3 to 4 strips and remove the seeds. Drain in a colander for about 30 minutes.

3. Add salt and pepper to taste only when ready to use. Drizzle with extra virgin olive oil. Serve.

TIPS

Only red and yellow peppers are used in this recipe. They are harvested from the same plant as the green ones, but are plumper and sweeter after changing color, since they are picked when fully ripe.

Roasted peppers can be stored in the refrigerator for up to 5 days or frozen for up to 6 months.

Variation

Grilled Peppers: Cut the peppers in half or into quarters, removing the seeds and ribs, then put them on an oiled baking sheet, turning to coat thoroughly with oil. Place the baking sheet under a preheated broiler, 3 to 4 inches (7.5 to 10 cm) from the heat, and cook for 5 to 6 minutes, turning once, until the peppers are soft and browned in spots. (Or arrange the peppers on a preheated barbecue grill and cook until golden brown, turning once.) Wrap the peppers in foil or a paper bag and let cool for a few minutes, then proceed with step 3.

Spinach with Raisins

**MAKES
4 SERVINGS**

Preparation time:

5 minutes

Cooking time:

10 minutes

TIP

Most nuts and seeds
are low-FODMAP when
eaten in amounts of
up to 2 tbsp (30 mL).
The only two nuts to
avoid at all costs are
pistachios and cashews.

1 lb	spinach (16 cups/4 L), trimmed	440 g
	Salt	
4 tsp	non-hydrogenated margarine	20 mL
4 tsp	pine nuts (optional)	20 mL
1 tbsp	raisins	15 mL

1. Wash and drain the spinach rapidly, then transfer to a pot or saucepan without adding any water. The water trapped in the leaves after gentle shaking is enough to cook them. Add salt, cover and cook over high heat for 3 to 4 minutes, until the leaves wilt and turn very deep green. Avoid overcooking; otherwise, the spinach will become brownish. Drain well.

2. Heat the margarine in a skillet over low heat. Add the cooked spinach, raisins and pine nuts (if using). Heat for 2 to 3 minutes, stirring often. Serve.

Vegan Variation
Substitute vegetable oil for the margarine.

NUTRIENTS PER SERVING	
Calories	60
Protein	3 g
Fat	4.5 g
Saturated fat	0.5 g
Carbohydrates	5 g
Fiber	2 g
Sodium	60 mg

Mint Zucchini

**MAKES
4 SERVINGS**

· MAKE AHEAD ·

Preparation time:

10 minutes

Cooking time:

20 minutes

*Here's a nice side dish
that can be converted to
a pasta sauce simply by
tossing it with pasta and
sprinkling with grated
Parmesan cheese.*

TIP

The zucchini can be
stored in the refrigerator
for up to 2 days.

2 tbsp	olive oil	30 mL
4	zucchini (1 lb, 2 oz/500 g total), cut into ½-inch (1 cm) pieces	4
	Salt	
⅓ cup	Allergen-Free Vegetable Broth (page 116)	75 mL
2 tbsp	finely chopped fresh mint	30 mL
	Freshly ground black pepper	

1. Heat the oil in a skillet over medium heat. Add the zucchini and cook, stirring occasionally, until the zucchini are softened and colored, about 8 to 10 minutes. Add a sprinkling of salt and sauté for 1 minute, stirring.

2. Turn the heat to low and add the broth. Cover and cook over low heat until the zucchini is very tender, 5 to 10 minutes. Stir in the mint, adjust the seasoning, then serve.

NUTRIENTS PER SERVING	
Calories	70
Protein	1 g
Fat	5.0 g
Saturated fat	0.5 g
Carbohydrates	5 g
Fiber	2 g
Sodium	35 mg

Greek-Style Roasted Vegetables

VEGAN

Preparation time:

15 minutes

Cooking time:

35 minutes

TIPS

Don't hesitate to add dry herbs to your recipes, to increase flavor without using garlic or onion.

The roasted vegetables can be stored in the refrigerator for up to 3 days.

• Preheat oven to 375°F (190°C)
• Baking sheet, generously oiled

2	parsnips	2
2	carrots	2
$\frac{1}{2}$	celeriac	$\frac{1}{2}$
2 tbsp	olive oil	30 mL
$1\frac{1}{2}$ tsp	dried oregano	7 mL
	Salt and freshly ground black pepper	

1. Peel the parsnips, carrots and celeriac, then cut them into uniform pieces approximately $\frac{3}{4}$ inch (2 cm) thick. Lay them out on the prepared baking sheet in one layer and coat thoroughly with the oil. Add the oregano. Season with salt and pepper to taste.

2. Roast in the middle of the preheated oven for about 35 to 40 minutes, until the vegetables are soft and golden-colored. Turn them twice during cooking. Serve.

NUTRIENTS PER SERVING	
Calories	120
Protein	2 g
Fat	5.0 g
Saturated fat	0.5 g
Carbohydrates	18 g
Fiber	4 g
Sodium	100 mg

Grilled Vegetables

**MAKES
4 SERVINGS**

· MAKE AHEAD ·

Preparation time:

10 minutes

Cooking time:

10 minutes

TIPS

If you can only find large eggplants (1 lb, 2 oz/ 500 g each or more), slice them either crosswise or lengthwise, sprinkle them with coarse salt, then let drain for about 30 minutes. Rinse well and pat dry. If the eggplants are small, this step is not necessary, as smaller eggplants are not bitter.

The grilled vegetables can be stored in the refrigerator for up to 3 days.

NUTRIENTS PER SERVING

Calories	130
Protein	3 g
Fat	9.0 g
Saturated fat	1.0 g
Carbohydrates	13 g
Fiber	5 g
Sodium	15 mg

- **Preheat barbecue grill to high or preheat broiler**
- **Baking sheet, oiled (if broiling)**

2	yellow or red bell peppers	2
4	zucchini (1 lb, 2 oz/500 g total)	4
2	small eggplants (13 oz/360 g total; see tip)	2
2 tbsp	olive oil	30 mL
	Salt and freshly ground black pepper	
1 tbsp	extra virgin olive oil	15 mL

1. If using an outdoor grill, cut the peppers in half and the zucchini and eggplant into about $2/3$-inch (1.5 cm) thick slices, for easier manipulation. Slice the zucchini lengthwise. (If using the broiler, cut the peppers into quarters and the other vegetables into $1/3$-inch/7 mm thick slices for reduced cooking time.)

2. Arrange the vegetables on the hot grill, brush generously with olive oil and sprinkle with plenty of salt and freshly ground pepper. Cook them until golden brown, turning once. The zucchini will take about 5 minutes to cook, the eggplant and peppers will take about 8 minutes. (Alternatively, put the vegetables on an oiled baking sheet, turning them to coat thoroughly with oil. Add salt and pepper. Broil $2^1/2$ to 4 inches/ 7 to 10 cm from the heat for about 3 minutes for the zucchini and eggplant, 5 minutes for the peppers.)

3. Peppers should be peeled before serving. To ease this operation, cover or wrap the peppers in foil or in a paper bag and let cool down a few minutes (the moisture kept under the cover will help lift the peel).

4. Serve the vegetables drizzled with extra virgin olive oil.

Mashed Potatoes

**MAKES
4 SERVINGS**

• **MAKE AHEAD** •

• **FREEZABLE** •

Preparation time:

10 minutes

Cooking time:

25 minutes

*Mashed potatoes make
for a great low-FODMAP
(and gluten-free) side dish.*

TIPS

A food mill or potato
ricer is very useful for
puréeing potatoes. A
food processor is not.

Mashed potatoes
can be stored in the
refrigerator for up to
3 days or frozen for
up to 3 months; thaw,
if necessary, before
reheating.

NUTRIENTS PER SERVING	
Calories	230
Protein	5 g
Fat	6.0 g
Saturated fat	1.0 g
Carbohydrates	40 g
Fiber	5 g
Sodium	55 mg

• **Food mill or potato ricer**

4	russet or yellow-fleshed potatoes (2 lbs, 3 oz/1 kg total)	4
2 tbsp	non-hydrogenated margarine	30 mL
$2/_3$ cup	unsweetened fortified almond milk (approx.)	150 mL
	Salt and freshly ground black pepper	

1. Wash the potatoes, leaving the skin on. Boil or steam until very tender, about 20 to 25 minutes. Drain well and peel.

2. Meanwhile, in a microwave-safe bowl, combine the almond milk with the margarine. Microwave on Medium-High (70%) power for about 10 seconds, until hot.

3. Pass the potatoes through a food mill and put the purée back into the pot used to cook them. Pour in the milk mixture. Add more or less milk depending on how creamy you like your purée. Season with salt and pepper to taste, then blend well using a spatula. Reheat and serve warm.

Vegan Variation

Substitute vegetable oil for the margarine.

Potato Purée with Olive Oil

MAKES 4 SERVINGS

· MAKE AHEAD ·

· FREEZABLE ·

Preparation time:

5 minutes

Cooking time:

25 minutes

If you find this purée too dense, just add some warm water.

TIP

Potato purée can be stored in the refrigerator for up to 3 days or frozen for up to 3 months; thaw, if necessary, before reheating.

NUTRIENTS PER SERVING	
Calories	180
Protein	2 g
Fat	10.0 g
Saturated fat	1.5 g
Carbohydrates	20 g
Fiber	2 g
Sodium	10 mg

- **Food mill or potato ricer (see tip, page 219)**

2	russet or yellow-fleshed potatoes (1 lb, 2 oz/500 g total)	2
4 tsp	freshly squeezed lemon juice	20 mL
3 tbsp	olive oil	45 mL
	Salt and freshly ground black pepper	

1. Wash the potatoes, leaving the skin on. Boil or steam until very tender, about 20 to 25 minutes. Drain well and peel.

2. Pass the potatoes through a food mill and put the purée back into the pot used to cook them. Add the lemon juice, olive oil and salt and pepper to taste. Blend well, using a spatula. Reheat and serve warm.

Rösti

**MAKES
4 SERVINGS**

Preparation time:

10 minutes

Cooking time:

15 minutes

*Originally a common
farmer's breakfast in the
canton of Bern, rösti has
become a national Swiss
specialty, eaten either
as a side dish or a main
course. There are many
variations of this popular
dish, using different
kinds of potatoes. In
some versions, the
potatoes are boiled before
they are grated. In its
homeland, rösti recipes
make for an interesting
subject of conversation!*

• **Preheat oven to 200°F (100°C)**

4	yellow-fleshed potatoes ($1\frac{3}{4}$ lbs/ 800 g total)	4
	Salt	
$\frac{1}{4}$ cup	butter	60 mL
$2\frac{1}{2}$ tbsp	olive oil (approx.)	38 mL

1. Peel the potatoes and grate them using a large-holed grater, without rinsing (the starch keeps the pancake together). Add salt.

2. Heat the butter and oil in a nonstick skillet over medium heat. Put one handful of the grated potatoes in the pan and press with a spatula to a thin layer, about $\frac{1}{3}$ inch (7 mm). (It is not important if the pancakes are imperfect in shape, but they must be thin, buttery and very crisp.) Continue to press while the rösti cooks so that it will stick together. Brown for 4 to 5 minutes until crisp on one side, then turn it over and brown for an additional 4 to 5 minutes, until crisp on the other side. You may need to add some more oil to the pan. When ready, set aside on a plate in a warm oven. Repeat for the remaining potato mixture. Serve.

Vegan Variation

Either use a vegan butter alternative or completely omit the butter. It will work either way!

NUTRIENTS PER SERVING	
Calories	270
Protein	3 g
Fat	15.0 g
Saturated fat	6.0 g
Carbohydrates	33 g
Fiber	3 g
Sodium	10 mg

Steamed Basmati Rice

**MAKES
4 SERVINGS**

· MAKE AHEAD ·

· FREEZABLE ·

Preparation time:

5 minutes

Cooking time:

15 minutes

Standing time:

5 minutes

*Basmati rice contains
more fiber and
nutrients than white
or instant rice.*

TIP

The cooked rice
can be stored in the
refrigerator for up to
2 days or frozen for
up to 3 months; thaw,
if necessary, before
reheating.

NUTRIENTS PER SERVING	
Calories	180
Protein	4 g
Fat	0.4 g
Saturated fat	0.1 g
Carbohydrates	40 g
Fiber	1 g
Sodium	2 mg

$2^3/_4$ cups	water	675 mL
$1^1/_3$ cups	basmati rice, rinsed and drained	325 mL
Pinch	salt	Pinch

1. Pour the water into a saucepan, cover and bring to a
   boil. Add the rice and salt. Cover and cook over very
   low heat for about 15 minutes, without uncovering.

2. Remove the saucepan from the heat. The water should
   be completely absorbed. If it isn't, cover and simmer
   for a few more minutes. Let stand, covered, for 3 to
   5 minutes. Serve.

Steamed Brown Rice

Preparation time:

5 minutes

Cooking time:

35 minutes

*Brown rice is more
nourishing and richer in
dietary fiber than white
rice. If you can find it,
buy brown Basmati rice,
which cooks in about half
the time and is fragrant.*

TIP

The cooked rice
can be stored in the
refrigerator for up to
2 days or frozen for
up to 3 months; thaw,
if necessary, before
reheating.

NUTRIENTS PER SERVING	
Calories	160
Protein	3 g
Fat	1.0 g
Saturated fat	0.2 g
Carbohydrates	33 g
Fiber	3 g
Sodium	2 mg

1 cup	long-grain brown rice, rinsed and drained	250 mL
2 cups	water	500 mL
Pinch	salt	Pinch

1. Pour the water into a saucepan, cover and bring to a boil. Add the rice and salt. Cover and cook over very low heat for about 35 minutes, without uncovering.

2. Remove the saucepan from the heat. The water should be completely absorbed. If it isn't, cover and simmer for a few more minutes. Serve.

Steamed Millet

MAKES 4 SERVINGS

· MAKE AHEAD ·

· FREEZABLE ·

Preparation time:

5 minutes

Cooking time:

25 minutes

Millet is an interesting alternative to rice. On top of being gluten-free and low-FODMAP, it is a great source of fiber.

TIP

The cooked millet can be stored in the refrigerator for up to 2 days or frozen for up to 3 months; thaw, if necessary, before reheating.

4 cups	water	1 L
1 cup	whole-grain hulled millet	250 mL
Pinch	salt	Pinch

1. Pour the water into a saucepan, cover and bring to a boil. Add the millet and salt. Cover and cook over very low heat for about 25 minutes, without uncovering.

2. Remove the saucepan from the heat. The water should be completely absorbed. If it isn't, cover and simmer for a few more minutes. Serve.

NUTRIENTS PER SERVING	
Calories	110
Protein	3 g
Fat	1.0 g
Saturated fat	0.2 g
Carbohydrates	23 g
Fiber	3 g
Sodium	2 mg

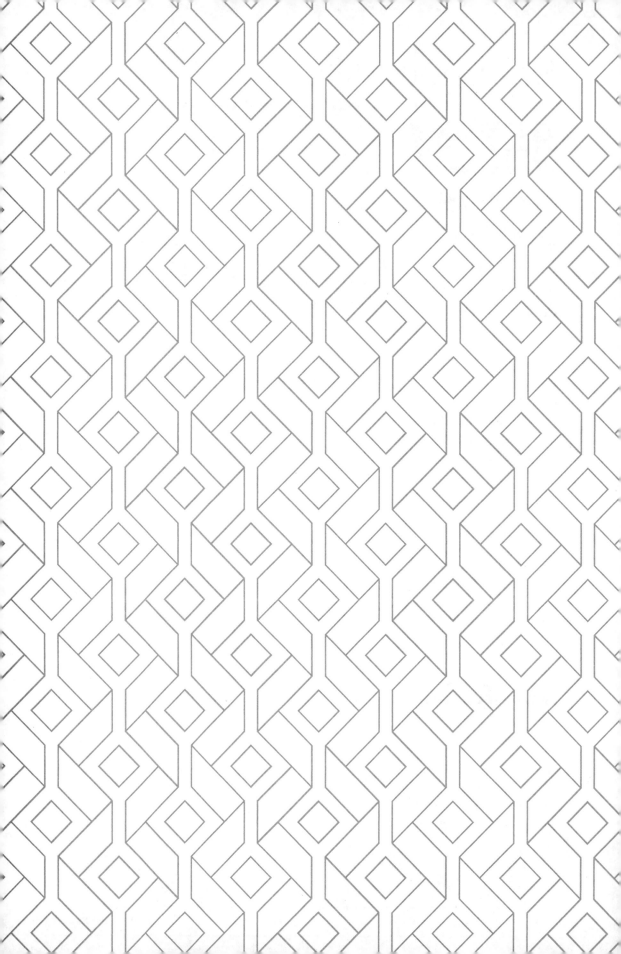

Desserts

Lemon Polenta Cake

VEGAN OPTION

Preparation time:

15 minutes

Cooking time:

30 minutes

Standing time:

1 hour

Vegan Variation

Swap the 3 eggs for 3 tbsp (45 mL) ground flax seeds (flaxseed meal) mixed with 1 cup (250 mL) water. Let the mixture rest for 5 minutes before adding it to the recipe, to allow it to gel.

NUTRIENTS PER SERVING

Calories	300
Protein	5 g
Fat	18.0 g
Saturated fat	1.5 g
Carbohydrates	32 g
Fiber	3 g
Sodium	55 mg

- Preheat oven to 350°F (180°C)
- Coffee grinder or mini chopper
- Electric mixer
- 10-inch (25 cm) springform pan, bottom lined with parchment paper, sides oiled

1 cup	granulated sugar	250 mL
1 cup	almonds	250 mL
½ cup	canola oil	125 mL
¾ cup	cornmeal (polenta)	175 mL
2 tsp	baking powder	10 mL
3	large eggs, beaten	3
	Juice of 2 lemons	
½ cup	confectioners' (icing) sugar	125 mL

1. Lightly grind the granulated sugar in a coffee grinder to make it just a bit finer, but not to confectioners' (icing) sugar consistency. Set aside in a bowl. Grind the almonds and set aside in another bowl.

2. In a large bowl, using the electric mixer, cream the ground sugar with the oil for about 5 minutes, until the mixture is pale and whipped. In another bowl, mix together the ground almonds, cornmeal and baking powder. Add the almond mixture to the sugar mixture, alternating with the eggs. Mix well until thoroughly blended.

3. Pour the mixture into the prepared cake pan and bake in the preheated oven for about 30 to 35 minutes. Check the cake with a toothpick or knife to see if it is cooked through. When done, pull the cake out of the oven and let it cool down in its pan.

4. Meanwhile, make the syrup. Mix together the lemon juice and confectioners' sugar in a microwave-safe measuring cup or bowl. Cook in a microwave on High, in 30-second intervals, until the sugar is dissolved into the juice.

5. Pour the warm syrup over the cake and let cool completely before taking it out of its pan. Serve.

Coconut Macaroons

MAKES 16 COOKIES

• **MAKE AHEAD** •

Preparation time:

10 minutes

Cooking time:

40 minutes

Standing time:

30 minutes

Macaroons are cookies that are crispy on the outside and chewy inside, and usually made of almond paste, sugar and egg whites. In this version, almond paste is replaced with coconut.

TIP

These cookies keep well in an airtight container at room temperature for up to 15 days.

NUTRIENTS PER SERVING	
Calories	50
Protein	1 g
Fat	2.0 g
Saturated fat	2.0 g
Carbohydrates	7 g
Fiber	1 g
Sodium	10 mg

• **Preheat oven to 300°F (150°C)**
• **Electric mixer**
• **Pastry bag or resealable plastic bag**
• **Large baking sheet, lined with parchment paper**

3	large egg whites	3
Pinch	salt	Pinch
³⁄₄ cup	confectioners' (icing) sugar	175 mL
²⁄₃ cup	unsweetened shredded coconut	150 mL

1. In a bowl, using the electric mixer, beat the egg whites and salt until stiff peaks form. Add the sugar gradually, 1 tbsp (15 mL) at a time, then continue to whip at high speed until the mixture is glossy and the sugar is dissolved, about 7 to 8 minutes. Fold in the coconut with a spatula.

2. Using either a pastry bag or a sealable plastic bag with a corner cut off (or simply a spoon), form small mounds (about 1 tbsp/15 mL of the mixture) on the prepared baking sheet. Leave about ¹⁄₂ inch (1 cm) of space between the macaroons.

3. Bake in the middle of the preheated oven for about 35 to 40 minutes, until the macaroons become light brown and can be removed easily from the paper. Let the macaroons cool down for about 30 minutes before serving.

Quinoa Pudding

**MAKES
6 SERVINGS**

• MAKE AHEAD •

• FREEZABLE •

Preparation time:

15 minutes

Cooking time:

1 hour

Nutritious quinoa is the star of this tasty dessert, which originates from Peru, where it is known as postre de quinoa.

- Fine-mesh sieve
- 9-inch (23 cm) square metal baking pan, oiled

1 cup	quinoa	250 mL
6 cups	water	1.5 L
3	large eggs	3
1 cup	unsweetened fortified almond milk	250 mL
1 tsp	vanilla extract	5 mL
¾ cup	granulated sugar	175 mL
	Salt	
½ cup	walnuts, chopped	125 mL
3 tbsp	raisins	45 mL
⅛ tsp	ground cinnamon	0.5 mL
½ cup	pure maple syrup (optional)	125 mL

1. Rinse quinoa in a sieve under running water and drain well. Bring quinoa and water to a boil in a large saucepan, then reduce heat and simmer, uncovered, until grains are translucent, 13 to 15 minutes. Drain well in the sieve. Set aside.

2. Meanwhile, preheat oven to 350°F (180°C).

3. In a large bowl, whisk together the eggs, milk, vanilla, all but 1 tbsp (15 mL) of the sugar and the salt until just combined. Stir in the cooked quinoa, nuts and raisins. Pour the mixture into the prepared pan.

4. In a small bowl, mix together the cinnamon and remaining sugar, then sprinkle on top of the pudding.

NUTRIENTS PER SERVING

Calories	260
Protein	7 g
Fat	7.0 g
Saturated fat	1.0 g
Carbohydrates	45 g
Fiber	2 g
Sodium	115 mg

The pudding can be wrapped and stored in the refrigerator for up to 3 days or frozen for up to 3 months; thaw, if necessary, before serving.

5. Bake in middle of oven for about 40 minutes or until a knife inserted in the center comes out clean. Serve warm or at room temperature, with maple syrup on the side, if desired.

Variation

Mini Quinoa Puddings: Instead of a baking pan, divide the quinoa mixture evenly among 6 small ramekins or a 6-cup silicon mold. Sprinkle with cinnamon sugar, dividing evenly. Reduce the baking time to about 30 minutes.

Vegan Variation

Replace the eggs with 3 tbsp (45 mL) ground flax seeds (flaxseed meal) mixed with 1 cup (250 mL) water. Let the mixture rest for 5 minutes before adding it to the recipe, to allow it to gel.

Tapioca Pudding

• MAKE AHEAD •

Preparation time:

10 minutes

Cooking time:

10 minutes

Standing time:

3 hours

TIPS

The egg white in this recipe is used raw. If the food safety of raw eggs is a concern for you, look for pasteurized liquid egg whites, sold in cartons in most grocery stores. Use 2 tbsp (30 mL) in this recipe.

Make sure you choose quick-cooking tapioca, which does not require soaking, nor a long cooking time.

NUTRIENTS PER SERVING

Calories	120
Protein	5 g
Fat	3.5 g
Saturated fat	2.5 g
Carbohydrates	18 g
Fiber	0 g
Sodium	120 mg

- Electric mixer

2 cups	lactose-free milk	500 mL
¼ cup	pearl tapioca (quick-cooking)	60 mL
¼ cup	granulated sugar	60 mL
¼ tsp	salt	1 mL
1	large egg (see tip)	1
3 tbsp	unsweetened coconut flakes	45 mL

1. Warm up the milk on the stovetop or in a microwave for 1 for 2 minutes, until lukewarm.

2. Add the tapioca, sugar and salt to a saucepan. Mix in the warmed milk. Cook over very low heat for 5 minutes, stirring.

3. Separate the egg white from the yolk. Put the egg white in a bowl and add the yolk to the saucepan. Cook for an additional 5 minutes over low heat, stirring. Remove the saucepan from the heat.

4. Beat the egg white to form stiff peaks using the electric mixer and fold them very gently into the tapioca mixture.

5. Portion out the pudding into small serving bowls (about ⅓ cup/75 mL each). Sprinkle with the coconut flakes. Chill for at least 3 hours in the refrigerator before serving.

Rice Pudding

**MAKES
4 SERVINGS**

• **MAKE AHEAD** •

Preparation time:

5 minutes

Cooking time:

1 hour

Standing time:

1 hour

*Most dried fruits are
high in FODMAPs.
However, in small
quantities, as in this
recipe, raisins are
usually well tolerated.*

TIP

Place plastic wrap on
top of the pudding to
prevent a skin from
forming and store in the
refrigerator for up to
2 days.

NUTRIENTS PER SERVING	
Calories	150
Protein	2 g
Fat	3.0 g
Saturated fat	0.0 g
Carbohydrates	33 g
Fiber	1 g
Sodium	130 mg

2 ¾ cups	unsweetened fortified almond milk	675 mL
⅓ cup	granulated sugar	75 mL
⅓ cup	Arborio rice	75 mL
1 tsp	vanilla extract	5 mL
¼ tsp	ground cinnamon	1 mL
2 tbsp	raisins	30 mL
3 tbsp	slivered almonds (optional)	45 mL

1. Bring the almond milk and sugar to a boil in a saucepan, then lower heat to medium. Almond milk must simmer but not boil.

2. Add rice to warm liquid. Stir well to prevent rice from sticking to pot. Keep heat to medium. Let simmer, stirring from time to time, for 60 minutes or until it thickens. Once cooked, remove from heat and stir in vanilla, cinnamon and raisins.

3. Let cool for at least 60 minutes, stirring from time to time, before serving. Add almonds (if using) just before serving.

Berry Tofu Mousse

Preparation time:

15 minutes

Standing time:

1 hour

A healthy and refreshing dessert.

TIP

The mousse can be stored in the refrigerator for up to 2 days or frozen for up to 2 months; thaw in the refrigerator, if necessary, before serving.

• **Blender**

14 oz	soft tofu	400 g
$1^2/_3$ cup	frozen raspberries or strawberries	400 mL
2 tsp	vanilla extract	10 mL
3 tbsp	pure maple syrup	45 mL
$1/_4$ cup	freshly squeezed lemon juice	60 mL
2 tbsp	unsweetened coconut flakes	30 mL

1. Put the tofu in the blender. Blend on maximum speed for about 1 minute, until smooth and creamy. Add the frozen berries, then blend until puréed. Add the vanilla extract, maple syrup and lemon juice. Blend well.

2. Pour the mixture into individual bowls. Chill the mousse in the refrigerator for about 1 hour before serving. Garnish each serving with coconut flakes and serve.

NUTRIENTS PER SERVING	
Calories	140
Protein	7 g
Fat	5.0 g
Saturated fat	2.0 g
Carbohydrates	21 g
Fiber	5 g
Sodium	15 mg

Kiwi and Orange Sabayon Gratin

Preparation time:

10 minutes

Cooking time:

15 minutes

A delicious dessert that must be prepared at the very last minute and eaten right away. Oranges, like most citrus fruits, are a great low-FODMAP choice.

- Preheat broiler
- Broiler-proof serving plates or dishes

2	kiwifruits	2
2	oranges	2
2	large egg yolks	2
2 tbsp	red wine	30 mL
1 tbsp	cold water	15 mL
3 tbsp	granulated sugar	45 mL
1 tbsp	confectioners' (icing) sugar	15 mL

1. Peel the kiwis and oranges, then slice them crosswise and place the slices on individual serving plates. Set aside.

2. To make the sabayon, put the yolks in a heatproof bowl. Pour in the red wine, cold water and granulated sugar. Set bowl over a saucepan of water over very low heat. Cook, whisking constantly, until thick and creamy, about 5 minutes. Portion out the sabayon over the fruit slices.

3. Put the plates in the oven as close to the upper heating element as possible and broil for about 2 to 3 minutes, until a golden crust has formed. Dust with confectioners' sugar and serve right away.

NUTRIENTS PER SERVING	
Calories	140
Protein	3 g
Fat	3.0 g
Saturated fat	1.0 g
Carbohydrates	25 g
Fiber	2 g
Sodium	5 mg

Papaya Cream

Preparation time:

10 minutes

A true Brazilian classic, at its best when freshly prepared. If you can't find lactose-free ice cream, use regular vanilla ice cream. Be sure not to increase the portion size.

TIPS

For best results, choose only a ripe papaya (yellow-skinned and yielding to gentle pressure).

Because papayas contain the enzyme papain, this cream does not keep well: prepare and eat it right away.

NUTRIENTS PER SERVING	
Calories	120
Protein	2 g
Fat	4.0 g
Saturated fat	2.5 g
Carbohydrates	20 g
Fiber	2 g
Sodium	25 mg

- **Blender**

½	ripe red papaya (about 1½ lbs/750 g)	½
4	scoops lactose-free vanilla ice cream (about 1 cup/250 mL total)	4

1. Cut the papaya in half lengthwise and remove the black seeds. Peel and discard the skin, which is not edible. Coarsely cut the pulp into pieces (about ⅔-inch/1.5 cm) and place them in a blender. Add the ice cream and pulse until very smooth.

2. Portion out the mixture into individual cups and serve immediately.

Quick Berry Sorbet

Preparation time:

15 minutes

Freezing time:

1 hour

TIPS

The egg white in this recipe is used raw. If the food safety of raw eggs is a concern for you, look for pasteurized liquid egg whites, sold in cartons in most grocery stores. One egg white equals 2 tbsp (30 mL) liquid egg whites.

The sorbet can be stored in the freezer for up to 1 week.

NUTRIENTS PER SERVING	
Calories	90
Protein	2 g
Fat	0.5 g
Saturated fat	0.0 g
Carbohydrates	20 g
Fiber	5 g
Sodium	15 mg

• **Blender**

2½ cups	frozen raspberries or strawberries (about 10½ oz/300 g)	625 mL
2 tsp	freshly squeezed lemon juice	10 mL
⅓ cup	confectioners' (icing) sugar	75 mL
1	large egg white (see tip)	1
	Fresh raspberries and/or strawberries	

1. Put the frozen berries in the blender. Add the lemon juice and confectioners' sugar, then blend on maximum speed. With the blender running, pour in the egg white and continue to mix until incorporated.

2. Transfer the mixture to a container, cover and chill in the freezer for at least 1 hour before serving. Garnish with a few berries and serve.

Ginger-Flavored Rhubarb Sorbet

**MAKES
6 SERVINGS**

· **MAKE AHEAD** ·

· **FREEZABLE** ·

Preparation time:

10 minutes

Cooking time:

15 minutes

Freezing time:

3 hours

TIP

After 7 to 10 days in the freezer, the sorbet will crystallize. To regain a smooth consistency, take the sorbet out of the freezer, bring it to room temperature, then repeat the stirring and freezing process.

NUTRIENTS PER SERVING	
Calories	120
Protein	1 g
Fat	0.2 g
Saturated fat	0.0 g
Carbohydrates	31 g
Fiber	1 g
Sodium	4 mg

5	stalks rhubarb (about 1 lb, 2 oz/500 g)	5
¾ cup	granulated sugar	175 mL
1½ tbsp	freshly squeezed lemon juice	22 mL
¾ cup	water	175 mL
1 tbsp	grated gingerroot	15 mL
1 tbsp	pure maple syrup (optional)	15 mL

1. Put a metal or glass bowl (or other freezer-safe container) in the freezer so that it will be cold when you fill it with the sorbet mixture.

2. Wash the rhubarb stalks briefly. Cut the stalks crosswise into approximately ⅔-inch (1.5 cm) pieces and set them aside.

3. Combine the sugar, lemon juice and water in a saucepan. Stir over low heat until the sugar dissolves, then bring to a boil and add the rhubarb. Lower the heat, cover and simmer for 8 to 10 minutes, until the rhubarb is tender.

4. Add the ginger to the saucepan. Cook for an additional 2 minutes and take the pan off the heat. If desired, add the maple syrup, which helps give the sorbet a velvety texture. Mix well.

5. Let the mixture cool down for about 10 minutes in the refrigerator, then pour it into the prepared container, cover and chill in the freezer. After about 2 hours, take the mixture out of the freezer and stir it with a whisk. Return it to the freezer and repeat the same stirring operation after another hour.

6. Take the sorbet out of the freezer for at least 15 minutes before serving, so that it will soften slightly.

Chocolate Fondue

**MAKES
4 SERVINGS**

· MAKE AHEAD ·

Preparation time:

15 minutes

Cooking time:

5 minutes

===

Make sure to use dark chocolate for this fondue. Not only will it taste better, but it ensures that the chocolate will not contain any added lactose (a FODMAP), which could cause symptoms.

TIP
You will need a fondue pot and burner to keep the chocolate warm. Each guest should have a dipping fork and a plate to let the chocolate cool a bit.

NUTRIENTS PER SERVING

Calories	460
Protein	5 g
Fat	29.0 g
Saturated fat	18.0 g
Carbohydrates	46 g
Fiber	5 g
Sodium	25 mg

- **Chocolate fondue set with candle**

³⁄₄ cup	lactose-free heavy or whipping (35%) cream (approx.)	175 mL
6¹⁄₃ oz	dark (70% cacao) chocolate	180 g
³⁄₄ cup	strawberries	175 mL
2	bananas, cut into rounds	2
2	clementines, segments separated	2
²⁄₃ cup	seedless grapes	150 mL

1. Pour the cream into a small pot, then heat over low heat until warm, but do not bring to a boil. Remove from heat, then add the chocolate. Let melt for 2 minutes, then stir, using a whisk, until the mixture becomes smooth.

2. Transfer to a fondue pot and put it on top of a burner. If the fondue is too thick for your taste, stir in some more cream (or your preferred liquor). Set out a tray of various fruits for your guests to dip in the fondue.

> **Vegan Variation**
> Substitute unsweetened almond milk or soy milk (from soy protein) for the lactose-free cream.

Small Bowl of Strawberries and Raspberries

VEGAN

Preparation time:

5 minutes

Standing time:

10 minutes

It's possible to swap either the strawberries or the raspberries for blueberries in this recipe. Don't choose blackberries, though, as they are high in FODMAPs!

¼ cup	strawberries	60 mL
¼ cup	raspberries	60 mL
1 tsp	freshly squeezed lemon juice	5 mL
½ tsp	granulated sugar	2 mL

1. Rinse the berries gently, without soaking them. Hull the strawberries and halve them lengthwise.

2. Put all the berries in a bowl, pour in the lemon juice, add the sugar and toss gently. Let stand for 10 minutes, then serve.

NUTRIENTS PER SERVING

Calories	40
Protein	1 g
Fat	0.3 g
Saturated fat	0.0 g
Carbohydrates	9 g
Fiber	3 g
Sodium	1 mg

Sugared Oranges

**MAKES
1 SERVING**

Preparation time:

5 minutes

Standing time:

10 minutes

You can use maple syrup instead of sugar in this recipe. Stay away from honey or agave syrup, as they are high in FODMAPs (excess fructose).

1	orange	1
1 tsp	freshly squeezed lemon juice	5 mL
$\frac{1}{2}$ tsp	granulated sugar	2 mL

1. Peel the orange and cut it into bite-size pieces. Put them in a bowl and sprinkle with lemon juice and sugar. Let rest for 10 minutes, then toss well and serve.

NUTRIENTS PER SERVING

Calories	70
Protein	1 g
Fat	0.2 g
Saturated fat	0.0 g
Carbohydrates	17 g
Fiber	2 g
Sodium	0 mg

Two-Colored Fruit Salad

Preparation time:

5 minutes

As tempting as fruit may be, keep your intake to no more than one portion per sitting. Even low-FODMAP fruits contain simple sugars, which can cause symptoms if consumed in large quantities.

½	kiwifruit	½
½	orange (blood orange, if available)	½
1½ tsp	freshly squeezed lemon juice	7 mL
½ tsp	granulated sugar	2 mL

1. Peel and slice the kiwi and orange into thin rounds. Arrange them on a flat dish so that they alternate and overlap slightly. Sprinkle with lemon juice and sugar. Serve.

NUTRIENTS PER SERVING

Calories	60
Protein	1 g
Fat	0.3 g
Saturated fat	0.0 g
Carbohydrates	16 g
Fiber	2 g
Sodium	1 mg

Acknowledgments

We would like to thank the hundreds of thousands of SOSCuisine.com subscribers for their loyalty, and particularly those who have subscribed to the low-FODMAP menus, launched in spring 2015, for their constant suggestions, which allow us to help people suffering from irritable bowel syndrome as effectively as possible.

Our thanks also go to Prof. Peter Gibson, MD, and Dr. Jane Muir, RD, of Monash University, for their support and encouragement.

References

Baumier M. Small intestinal bacterial overgrowth. Today's Dietitian, 2015 Jul; 17 (7): 50. Available at: www.todaysdietitian.com/newarchives/070115p50.shtml.

Bolen B. The worst things to say to someone who has IBS [blog post]. Updated May 20, 2016. Available at: www.verywell.com/unhelpful-advice-for-ibs-1944712.

Canadian Nutrient File (2012). Retrieved June 15, 2015, from http://webprod3.hc-sc.gc.ca/cnf-fce/start-debuter.do?lang=fra.

Catsos P. FODMAPs and soy: Why so confusing? [blog post]. May 18, 2014. Available at: www.ibsfree.net/news/2014/5/18/fodmaps-and-soy-why-so-confusing?rq=soy.

Chey WD, Kurlander J, Eswaran S. Irritable bowel syndrome: A clinical review. *JAMA*, 2015; 313 (9): 949–58.

Ciorba MA. A gastroenterologist's guide to probiotics. *Clin Gastroenterol Hepatol*, 2012 Sep; 10 (9): 960–68.

Clairmont S. How to cope with IBS on vacation [blog post]. January 10, 2016. Available at: www.stephanieclairmont.com/how-to-cope-with-ibs-on-vacation.

Di Cagno R, De Angelis M, Lavermicocca P, et al. Proteolysis by sourdough lactic acid bacteria: Effects on wheat flour protein fractions and gliadin peptides involved in human cereal intolerance. *Appl Environ Microbiol*, 2002 Feb; 68 (2): 623–33.

Dietitians of Canada and PEN — Practice-based Evidence in Nutrition. Healthy eating guidelines for irritable bowel syndrome [article in French]. December 30, 2015. Available at: www.pennutrition.com/viewhandout.aspx?Portal=UbY=&id=JMznUQY=&PreviewHandout=bA==.

El-Seraq HB. Impact of irritable bowel syndrome: Prevalence and effect on health-related quality of life. *Rev Gastroenterol Disord*, 2003; 3 Suppl 2: S3–11.

Gibson PR, Shepherd SJ. (2010). Evidence-based dietary management of functional gastrointestinal symptoms: The FODMAP approach. *J Gastroenterol Hepatol*, 2009 Oct 14; 25 (2): 252–58.

Gibson PR, Varney J, Malakar S, Muir JG. Food components and irritable bowel syndrome. *Gastroenterol*, 2015 May; 148 (6): 1158–74.

Greco L, Gobbetti M, Auricchio R, et al. Safety for patients with celiac disease of baked goods made of wheat flour hydrolyzed during food processing. *Clin Gastroenterol Hepatol*, 2011 Jan; 9 (1): 24–29.

Halmos EP, Christophersen CT, Bird AR, et al. Diets that differ in their FODMAP content alter the colonic luminal microenvironment. *Gut*, 2015; 64 (1): 93–100.

Irritable Bowel Syndrome Self Help and Support Group. About irritable bowel syndrome: IBS explained for people who do not have IBS [blog post]. Updated January 4, 2011. Available at: www.ibsgroup.org/aboutibs.

Leblanc N. L'impact des macronutriments et des fibres sur le SII [PowerPoint presentation in French]. April 27, 2014. Available at: http://www.harmoniesante.com/HS/formations/Formation_114_1_Partie_2_Impact_macronutriments_fibres_SII_Fodmap.pdf.

Mansueto P, Seidita A, D'Alcamo A, Carroccio A. Role of FODMAPs in patients with irritable bowel syndrome. *Nutr Clin Pract*, 2015 Oct; 30 (5): 665–82.

Marsh A, Eslick EM, Eslick GD. Does a diet low in FODMAPs reduce symptoms associated with functional gastrointestinal disorders? A comprehensive systematic review and meta-analysis. *Eur J Nutr*, 2016 Apr; 55 (3): 897–906.

Monash University. The Monash University Low FODMAP Diet (Version 1.4) [mobile app]. 2015 Downloaded from http://itunes.apple.com.

Muir J. Are all spelt products low in FODMAPs? [blog post]. Monash University. April 1, 2015. Available at: fodmapmonash. blogspot.ca/2015/03/are-all-spelt-products-low-in-fodmaps.html.

Muir JG, Rose R, Rosella O, et al. Measurement of short-chain carbohydrates in common Australian vegetables and fruits by high-performance liquid chromatography (HPLC). *J Agric Food Chem*, 2009; 57 (2): 554–65.

Pimentel M, Morales W, Rezaie A, et al. Development and validation of a biomarker for diarrhea-predominant irritable bowel syndrome in human subjects. *PLoS ONE*, 2015 May 13; 10 (5): e0126438.

Rezaie A, Pimentel M, Rao SS. How to test and treat small intestinal bacterial overgrowth: An evidence-based approach. *Curr Gastroenterol Rep*, 2016 Jan 16; 18 (2): 8.

Rizello CG, De Angelis M, Di Cagno R, et al. Highly efficient gluten degradation by lactobacilli and fungal proteases during food processing: New perspectives for celiac disease. *Appl Environ Microbiol*, 2007 Jul; 73 (14): 4499–507.

Scarlata K. Small intestinal bacterial overgrowth (SIBO) [blog post]. January 22, 2014. Available at: blog.katescarlata.com/2014/01/22/small-intestinal-bacterial-overgrowth.

Scott A. Confused about soy & the low FODMAP diet? [blog post]. Updated June 20, 2016. Available at: www.alittlebityummy.com/blog/confused-about-soy-and-the-low-fodmap-diet.

Shepherd S, Gibson P. *The Complete Low-FODMAP Diet: A Revolutionary Plan for Managing IBS and Other Digestive Disorders*. New York: The Experiment, 2013.

Shepherd SJ, Lomer MCE, Gibson PR. Short-chain carbohydrates and functional gastrointestinal disorders. *Am J Gastroenterol*, 2013; 108 (5): 707–17.

Shepherd SJ, Parker FC, Muir JG, Gibson PR. Dietary triggers of abdominal symptoms in patients with irritable bowel syndrome: Randomized placebo-controlled evidence. *Clin Gastroenterol Hepatol*, 2008 Jul; 6 (7): 765–71.

Staudacher HM, Whelan K, Irving PM, Lomer MCE. Comparison of symptom response following advice for a diet low in fermentable carbohydrates (FODMAPs) versus standard dietary advice in patients with irritable bowel syndrome. *J Hum Nutr Diet*, 2011 Oct; 24 (5): 487–95.

Tuck C. Avoiding wheat — How strict on a low FODMAP diet? [blog post]. Monash University. August 10, 2015. Available at: fodmapmonash.blogspot.ca/2015/08/avoiding-wheat-how-strict-on-low-fodmap.html.

Varney J. Talking tofu [blog post]. Monash University. December 10, 2015. Available at: fodmapmonash.blogspot.ca/2015/12/talking-tofu.html.

Trustworthy Internet Resources

SOSCuisine.com

Personalized low-FODMAP recipes and meal plans: www.soscuisine.com/low-fodmap

One-on-one consultations with registered dietitians specializing in the low-FODMAP diet: www.soscuisine.com/low-fodmap/#tab3

Blog: www.soscuisine.com/blog/tag/fodmap-en

Monash University

Website: www.med.monash.edu/cecs/gastro/fodmap

Blog: fodmapmonash.blogspot.ca

App for Android and iPhone: http://www.med.monash.edu/cecs/gastro/fodmap/iphone-app.html

Canadian Society of Intestinal Research

Website: www.badgut.org

How to Find a Dietitian Who Specializes in FODMAP

VIP Personal Dietitian Service from SOSCuisine.com: www.soscuisine.com/low-fodmap/#tab3

Dietitians of Canada: www.dietitians.ca/Your-Health/Find-A-Dietitian

Academy of Nutrition and Dietetics: www.eatright.org/find-an-expert

British Dietetic Association: www.bda.uk.com/improvinghealth/yourhealth/finddietitian

FODMAP Registered Dietitian Registry, US & Canada: www.katescarlata.com/fodmapdietitians

Apps and Websites to Find Available Bathrooms

Sit or Squat
Bathroom Map
GoHere

Library and Archives Canada Cataloguing in Publication

Cuneo, Cinzia, 1956-
[Solution FODMAP. English]
   The low-FODMAP solution : put an end to IBS symptoms and abdominal pain /
Cinzia Cuneo, MSc and the Nutrition Team at SOSCuisine.com.

Includes index.
Translation of: La solution FODMAP.
ISBN 978-0-7788-0569-4 (softcover)

   1. Irritable colon—Nutritional aspects. 2. Irritable colon—Diet therapy.
3. Irritable colon—Diet therapy—Recipes. 4. Cookbooks. I. Title. II. Title: Solution FODMAP. English.

RC862.I77L6913 2017   616.3'42   C2017-901035-2

About SOSCuisine.com

SOSCuisine, active since 2005, is the website of choice for intelligent meal plans and grocery shopping planning for people with specific nutritional needs. Our meal plans are an efficient prevention and maintenance tool for several medical and nonmedical conditions. They are based on proven evidence relating to human nutrition and are constantly updated by our team of registered dietitians. SOSCuisine.com is recommended by many health sector bodies, including the University of Montreal's Health Centre, the Montreal Heart Institute's EPIC Center, the Médecins Francophones du Canada, the Canadian Society of Intestinal Research and the Quebec Foundation for Celiac Disease.

SOSCuisine.com offers meal plans and recipes adapted to those who have specific needs associated with health problems (metabolic, cardiovascular, gastrointestinal, etc.), are at certain points of life (pregnancy, menopause, etc.) or have personal goals (weight loss, marathon, hockey, etc.). All of the meal plans are based on the Mediterranean diet, which has proven benefits and is advocated by the Montreal Heart Institute's EPIC Center.

More than 400,000 families already use SOSCuisine.com to make intelligent dietary choices that are adapted to their needs, thanks to the variety of balanced meal plans that take into account people's dietary preferences and take advantage of the discounts announced by Canadian supermarkets. The service is offered in English, French and Italian.

About the Authors

Cinzia Cuneo
Cofounder and CEO of Sukha Technologies Inc.
Italian by birth and Canadian by adoption, Cinzia (pronounced "chin-tsia") decided to combine her professional experience and her passion for good food by developing a service that would help the many people who need to regain control of their diet. An engineer by training (chemical engineering, Polytechnic University of Turin, Italy), Cinzia holds a Master's in Applied Sciences from Polytechnique Montreal. She has traveled and lived in several countries while pursuing a demanding career within multinationals in the high-tech industry. In 2005, Cinzia founded Sukha Technologies, the company that developed and operates the website SOSCuisine.com.

The SOSCuisine Nutrition Team
Our dietitians dedicate themselves body and soul to improving your diet so that you can achieve your goals. They use new technologies to simplify your life and offer you a highly personalized service. Thanks to the computerized decision support system developed by SOSCuisine, they automatically generate your meal plans and grocery lists based on *your* wants and needs, while ensuring that they respect the most recent applicable recommendations. They take advantage of our blog and social networks to help you develop a diet that's truly adapted to your situation. In brief, each day they innovate a little more so that it becomes child's play for you to apply the diet that suits you best, whatever that may be (gluten-free, low-FODMAP, etc.)!

Danielle Lamontagne

Registered Dietitian, Director of the Nutrition Team
Member of the Ordre Professionnel des Diététistes du Québec
(OPDQ), with 25 years of experience, Danielle has led the
Nutrition Team since 2006. Her expertise in personalized
diet reprogramming, a method to encourage people to make
conscious and sustainable changes, is an integral part of the
SOSCuisine formula. Danielle has been present at each stage
of the creation of the low-FODMAP meal plan to manage and
steer this large-scale project.

Jef L'Ecuyer

Registered Dietitian
A member of the OPDQ and Dietitians of Canada, Jef offers
a simple, effective and practical look at daily meal planning.
She dove into the universe of low-FODMAP nutrition as soon
as she arrived at SOSCuisine in January 2015. Thanks to her
passion for the culinary arts, she has been able to adapt the
SOSCuisine recipes to reduce their FODMAP content while
preserving their flavor.

Éloïse Vincent

Dietetic Technician and Gastronome
A member of our SOSCuisine team since 2009, Éloïse holds
the rare diploma of "Gastronome" from the University of
Gastronomic Sciences in Italy. She is also a dietetic technician.
During this book's creation, Éloïse was in charge of quality-
controlling the nutritional calculations and coordinating
the photographers so that the SOSCuisine recipes look as
beautiful as they are delicious.

Index